Supporting Autistic People Through Pregnancy and Childbirth

T0385259

of related interest

Supporting Survivors of Sexual Abuse
Through Pregnancy and Childbirth
A Guide for Midwives, Doulas and Other Healthcare Professionals
Kicki Hansard
Forewords by Penny Simkin and Phyllis Klaus
ISBN 978 1 84819 424 3
eISBN 978 0 85701 377 4

Stretched to the Limits
A Guide for Midwives and Doulas when Supporting Women with
EDS Through Pregnancy, Labour, Birth and Postnatally
Rachel Fitz-Desorgher
ISBN 978 1 83997 249 2
eISBN 978 1 83997 250 8

Supporting Autistic People Through Pregnancy and Childbirth

**HAYLEY MORGAN, EMMA DURMAN
AND KAREN HENRY**

Forewords by Carly Jones, Wenn B. Lawson
and Sheena Byrom

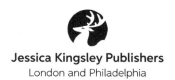

Jessica Kingsley Publishers
London and Philadelphia

First published in Great Britain in 2024 by Jessica Kingsley Publishers
An imprint of John Murray Press

1

Copyright © Hayley Morgan, Emma Durman and Karen Henry 2024

The right of Hayley Morgan, Emma Durman and Karen Henry to be
identified as the Authors of the Work has been asserted by them in
accordance with the Copyright, Designs and Patents Act 1988.

Foreword copyright © Carly Jones 2024
Foreword copyright © Wenn B. Lawson 2024
Foreword copyright © Sheena Byrom 2024

A CIP catalogue record for this title is available from the
British Library and the Library of Congress

ISBN 978 1 83997 105 1
eISBN 978 1 83997 106 8

Printed and bound by CPI Group (UK) Ltd, Croydon, CR0 4YY

Jessica Kingsley Publishers' policy is to use papers that are natural, renewable
and recyclable products and made from wood grown in sustainable
forests. The logging and manufacturing processes are expected to conform
to the environmental regulations of the country of origin.

Jessica Kingsley Publishers
Carmelite House
50 Victoria Embankment
London EC4Y 0DZ

www.jkp.com

John Murray Press
Part of Hodder & Stoughton Ltd
An Hachette Company

Contents

Foreword by Carly Jones

When Jessica Kingsley Publishers emailed me to ask if I'd add a foreword to *Supporting Autistic People Through Pregnancy and Childbirth* it felt like a pinch-me moment.

This was not only because the authors, such esteemed professionals, would consider me worthy of that privilege, but also because this is the book the NHS, wider international healthcare and autistic people themselves have been waiting for with baited breath for years, indeed, decades.

As co-production lead for the NHS in the Learning Disabilities and Autism programme in London I immediately invited one of the authors (who I feel should now at all times be referred to as the Charlie's Angels of autistic people and pregnancy) to speak to our NHS autism community of practice on this subject matter – subject which despite being mostly overlooked historically is now thankfully being given the systematic awareness it so richly deserves and requires.

Their talk had an impact beyond our imagination. With national films about autistic pregnancy now well under way, it feels like we are carefully yet confidently tiptoeing into a new era of support, understanding and non-infantilised equality for autistic people at a most pivotal time, that of becoming a parent.

Some weeks later I received hot off the press the final draft, which you as a reader have the honour of holding in your hands right now.

Carving out a full day in one of the admittedly rare sunshine-filled days here in the UK, I took to my garden and inhaled their collective words like a continuous breath of fresh air and deep exhalation of 'at last', nodding with agreement at every page I read.

Issues that are all too often overlooked that affect autistic pregnant people are explained, such as pain and interoception (hurrah at blinking last!), and the myth of autism and high intelligence meaning we have no care needs burst wide open with my favourite quote of the book, 'How can you be so intelligent but have no common sense?', which I'll add is a quote I heard often pre-diagnosis...and admittedly a few times after! What a contrast to the past, not so distant at all.

In 2014 I was fortunate enough to be an advisor for a Cambridge University study on autistic motherhood. The conclusion then was that autistic pregnant people were often so misunderstood by professionals that one in five were subject to social services interventions. In 2016 when acting as a research participant for an American university study on autistic people in childbirth I discovered that, anecdotally, our access to equitable pain relief and understanding of our emotional state post birth were also indirectly compromised.

Supporting Autistic People Through Pregnancy and Childbirth offers a candid, well thought out, factual and objective read that's written in such a manner that you can binge-read it in one sitting (as I did) or use as an on-hand reference guide with easy-to-locate sections as a go-to resource in practice.

Supporting Autistic People Through Pregnancy and Childbirth is more than another autism book; it's an invaluable record of the many vast experiences pregnant autistic people have faced and have tried to explain, to those who ask, for decades.

When asked 'What hurdles do autistic people have in pregnancy?', before now I'd sigh, 'Oh my gosh, how long do you have and where do I start?'

Now, I'll simply smile, and hand them a copy of this powerful book.

You'll leave this book feeling educated, with many 'aha!' moments and with a new-found hope that the next generation of autistic pregnant people will be less misunderstood and more hopeful.

Thank you, Hayley, Emma and Karen for all you do and for assisting the many people this will continue to help.

Dr Carly Jones MBE, h(DS)c

Foreword by Wenn B. Lawson

For autistic 'mums', childbearers, the medical community and others who support the birthing process as well as wanting to understand us, this book is so important and so very much needed. As an autistic 'mum' myself who birthed four children over four decades ago, I had very little understanding of what to expect. I read as much as I could about pregnancy (diet, exercise and so on) and about breastfeeding and motherhood, but all the information was for allistic or non-autistic individuals and our ways of processing and interacting with the world are so different. So, in many ways nothing prepared me, an autistic neurodivergent individual, for giving birth, my pain and how I would feel afterwards.

My first labour experience was very painful and very long, not unusual. I was induced, again not unusual, but the information given was sadly lacking, let alone offered in ways that might make sense for me as an autistic person. So, not being prepared for the experience – what it meant to have an episiotomy, the pain and the attitude of the attending midwife ('people have been having babies for thousands of years, it can't be that bad, now stop making such a fuss...') – was extremely traumatic. In the end the sedation used caused me to be totally 'out of it'. When I came to and asked about my baby, I was told that he was fine and in the nursery, and that I would see him the next morning. I remember thinking that wasn't what I expected and was very surprised and unhappy. I had read that 'baby' should be put to the breast after birth and there was no need to separate mother and child. (This separation was common in the 1970s; thankfully things have changed.)

But 'being and feeling' these things didn't mean I could easily convert these feelings into awareness and voice them. I worried very much about how my son was being fed and what was happening to him. When I finally got to see him the next day, I was also surprised that I didn't have any specific 'feeling' towards him. I mean, in the films and on television mothers cried as they held their newborn. But I didn't feel like crying. I only felt a kind of detachment and a strangeness.

Looking back over that time and subsequent times for my further three births over eight years between 1974 and 1982, some things changed heaps. But the one thing that didn't change for me was not having my voice and needs taken seriously. For example, I needed to 'do' practical care for my baby. I couldn't learn how to change a nappy, bathe a newborn and hold them from watching someone else do it. There is quite a bit of literature that suggests autistics are visual learners. But not me! I'm an auditory and kinesthetic learner despite having auditory processing disorder. Having our sensory needs accommodated before and as we go into labour is a must for autistic people. We need medical teams to understand autism and to listen to the autistic individual's words of apprehension, fear and even panic at times.

There will also be those among our ranks who will not connect to their birthing experience due to our interoception disconnection. There will be others who almost 'over connect' for similar reasons. All their monotropic [single-focused] attention will be in one place, possibly heightening certain experiences and being completely taken up with these.

There is a pervasive stereotype (thanks to Theory of Mind (ToM) arguments) that autistic people lack empathy, but this is misleading and far from true. In fact, thanks to monotropism, all too often we almost 'over feel' things and can become completely depleted in energy that is taken up by the expulsion of 'feeling' too much for others. This is essential to understand when working to support autistic future mums and childbearers.

Being 'mono' also means an individual doesn't divide attention easily, which can be a barrier to comprehending signals from our other senses (both external and internal).

As an autistic person I am single-minded, so it's more likely I'm not noticing something someone is pointing out to me due to my attending elsewhere. It can seem I lack understanding of other's mental states because my attention is occupied by what I'm interested in. It's not a lack of empathy but it might mean missing the signs that point toward an empathic understanding. Once these dots are joined up, I am as capable of empathy as the next person.

Very often when I utilise my interests to connect me to the bigger picture through role play, technology, story, objects, TV, YouTube and so on I'll connect more readily because these capture my interest, and therefore they capture my attention.

When I am focused it is like those things are highlighted by a narrow torch beam that means I am enveloped by my interests or passions, which I am connected to. But I can adjust to my environment and physical, emotional and cognitive states, I can learn, but I need to begin with where my interest is. So, to prevent me being disconnected, please capture my attention using concepts within my interests and passions.

Figuratively speaking, as described earlier, allistics are using the wider beam of a torch to grasp more context and connection across wider attended points, whereas an autistic person is using the bright narrow beam of a torch.

As autistic individuals the following points are crucial to understanding what might be happening for us as we travel through our pregnancy experience and deliver our babies.

- **Literality** (e.g. literal meaning of words, sentences, idioms, situations, forms of expression, feelings and so on). Difficulty understanding allegorical language.

- **Thinking in closed concepts** (e.g. staying with rules, habits, expectations, resistance to change, not understanding or finishing an incomplete sentence).

- **Context and scale** (e.g. difficulty generalising things, situations or learning).

- **Timing, sequencing and predicting** (e.g. difficulties in organising timings, intentions or the completion of various tasks, forward-thinking and appreciating outcomes may only occur in connection to interest).

- **Non-social priorities** (e.g. preferring casual wear that one has grown fond of or feels comfortable in rather than fashion or the need to dress for specific occasions).

As you read this book please keep these concepts in mind and take on board the learnings that can help in developing the important understanding that autistic individuals need you to consider as you support us.

Dr Wenn B. Lawson, PhD

References and resources

American Psychiatric Association (2013). *Diagnostic and Statistical Manual of Mental Disorders (DSM-5)*. Arlington, VA: APA.

Ashinoff, B.K. & Abu-Akel, A. (2021). Hyperfocus: The forgotten frontier of attention. *Psychological Research 85*(1):1–19.

Goodall, E. (2016). Thriving at school: How interoception is helping children and young people engage in learning every day. University of Southern Queensland, Toowoomba, Australia.

Gomot, M., Belmonte, M.K., Bullmore, E.T., Bernard, F.A. & Baron-Cohen, S. (2008). Brain hyper-activity to auditory novel targets in children with high-functioning autism. *Brain 131*(9), 2479–2488.

Kohli, J.S., Kinnear, M.K., Fong, C.H., Fishman, I. *et al.* (2019). Local cortical gyrification is increased in children with autism spectrum disorders, but decreases rapidly in adolescents. *Cerebral Cortex 29*(6), 2412–2423.

Lawson, W.B. & Dombroski, B.A. (2015). Might we be calling problems seen in autism spectrum conditions: 'poor theory of mind', when actually they are related to non-generalised 'object permanence'? *Journal of Intellectual Disability – Diagnosis and Treatment 3*(1), 43–48.

Lawson, W.B. & Dombroski, B.A. (2017). Problems with object permanence: Rethinking traditional beliefs associated with poor theory of mind in autism. *Journal of Intellectual Disability – Diagnosis and Treatment 5*(1), 1–6.

Lawson, W. (1998). *Life Behind Glass.* NSW, Australia: Southern Cross University Press.

Lawson, W. (2002). *Autism and Attention.* Good Autism Practice.

Lawson, W. (2011). *The Passionate Mind: How People with Autism Learn.* London: Jessica Kingsley Publishers.

Lawson, W. (2013). Sensory connection, interest/attention and gamma synchrony in autism or autism, brain connections and preoccupation. *Medical Hypotheses 80*(3), 284–288.

Mottron, L., Dawson, M., Soulières, I., Hubert, B., & Burack, J.A. (2006). Enhanced perceptual functioning in autism: An updated model and eight principles of autistic perception. *Journal of Autism and Developmental Disorders 36*(1), 27–43.

Murray, D., Lesser, M. & Lawson, W. (2005). Attention, monotropism and the diagnostic criteria for autism. *Autism 9*(2), 139–156.

Rusting, R. (2018). Decoding the overlap between autism and ADHD. *Spectrum News*, 7 February. https://doi.org/10.53053/KCZY8213.

Foreword by Sheena Byrom

In their busy and often challenging day-to-day lives, midwives and other professionals working in maternity care are tasked with providing personalised maternity care, which means approaching and caring for each childbearing woman and person as an individual. This can only happen when staff have a broad and in-depth understanding of different social and cultural backgrounds and of diversity in its entirety, all of which inform the needs and preferences of the people they serve. Pregnancy and childbirth is a time of life-change and affects us all; we are all born. Those with extra needs often face a double vulnerability when inequalities exist due to lack of awareness or judgement. How women, birthing people and families are treated during their childbearing journey influences outcomes both physical and psychological. What we do, and how we do it, what we say, and how we say it, matters. And this is critical for those we work with too.

We live in a world that continually unfolds with diverse human experiences, where we can learn about, embrace and celebrate neurodiversity. This book on supporting autistic people through pregnancy and childbirth offers enlightenment by inviting readers on a journey of understanding, compassion and appreciation to enhance health and wellbeing for birthing parents and their babies.

As healthcare professionals it is imperative that we are continually self-reflective, aware of our inbuilt and learned biases and that we continuously expand our knowledge to enhance our understanding and appreciation. I have learned so much from this exceptional text. Even as an experienced midwife of many decades each chapter made me sit up and re-read sentences – especially around the reality of the stigma autistic people face and the disrespectful attitudes due to lack of awareness.

I have a specific interest in the promotion of compassionate maternity care and compassionate leadership, so the content has provided me with another layer of knowledge to inform my work. Promoting safety in maternity services is crucial but often limited to risk management strategies and excessive monitoring of clinical situations and processes. However, evidence tells us that safe services are those where managers and leaders foster supportive, inclusive work environments and psychosocial safety is a priority. This is especially important when considering the needs of autistic people in their working and birthing environments, extra considerations for self-care (staff), how we communicate and the impact of empathy.

This book is a heartfelt and illuminating exploration of a subject that has long been shrouded in mystery and misunderstanding. From beginning to end the content is rich with information derived from a combination of lived experience, evidence-based and practice-based knowledge which the authors hope will open minds and hearts to the specific needs of autistic people – of both those working in and using maternity services.

Through these pages, you will gain insight into the everyday struggles and triumphs of autistic people who are on the journey of creating a family. This book is not just an opportunity to learn; it is an invitation to empathise, to embrace differences and to champion inclusivity. It is a call to action for a world that is more compassionate, more understanding and more accessible for all.

I am honoured to introduce you to this book, and I am confident that it will not only inform but also inspire you to join the journey towards a world where autism is not something to be feared or fixed but celebrated and supported.

So, open these pages and read on – within them lies a bank of evidence-based knowledge as well as a tapestry of stories, and hope that has the power to transform lives and perceptions.

Sheena Byrom OBE, Univ., Ed D honoris causa, RM, MA

About This Book

This work explores the specific needs of autistic mothers and childbearers during pregnancy, birth and transition to parenthood.

Born from personal experience and reinforced by wider anecdotal accounts, the need for tailored support for autistic mothers and childbearers in maternity care is discussed through a review of the wider literature base and current practices.

As a result of the identified needs, this resource includes a toolkit of strategies for midwives, maternity and wider healthcare professionals, with an aim to increase understanding of the specific needs of autistic mothers and childbearers during pregnancy, childbirth and new motherhood. The ultimate aim here is to improve experiences through the provision of tailored, empathetic, insightful care.

.

Author Biographies

Hayley Morgan, BA, PGCE, MSc

Hayley Morgan is an autistic mother and academic. Her passion is that of promoting equality of identity and self and access to healthcare for autistic parents. She began her journey writing about being autistic and pregnant with online Irish magazine *The M Word*. Her two articles about miscarriage, pregnancy and settling into life as a mum just at the time of diagnosis became a hugely rewarding pastime.

Hayley has presented at PARC London South Bank University, once alone about the relationship between protodeclarative gestures and empathy in autism, and a second time with Emma about the autistic birth experience. Hayley has previously delivered seminars with Autside Training and Consultancy, including Autism and Sensory Differences, Autism and Communication, Autism and Behaviour of Concern, Autism and Anxiety, and Teen Life modules. Hayley also worked with Autside to deliver to frontline staff including counter-terrorism police.

Hayley is currently completing a PhD in Human and Health Sciences at Swansea University, focusing on the autistic birth experience and the narratives of those involved in their care.

Emma Durman, MSc

Emma is a late-diagnosed autistic woman, with multiple co-occurring conditions, and is mother to an autistic transgender teenager. She is co-director of Autside Education and Training, a company that specialises in training, consultancy and support for a wide range of families and professionals across the public, private and third sectors. Clients include local authorities, Integrated Autism Services, Heathrow Airport, Home Office/WECTU (Welsh Counter-Terrorism Unit) and a range of social housing providers for which she received a commendation from the WECTU and a national Welsh Housing Award in collaboration with Mi-Space, a contractor that specialises in social housing renovations and improvements. Emma has also worked closely with the Welsh government via Autism Wales and the Integrated Autism Services on a range of issues, including being part of several writing and technical groups, also working to diversify and provide support and guidance throughout the Covid-19 pandemic. She was intrinsic to the creation of the recently launched Welsh Government Guidance on Autism and Housing and has delivered training and content to a variety of community of practice and neurodevelopmental conferences on several topics relating to autism, including pregnancy and parenthood. Emma has spoken at a variety of conferences in the UK and Europe and has been a coordinator on a pan-European Erasmus+ project on autism and employment alongside the National Autistic Society.

Emma focused her dissertation on the autistic birth experience, specifically on a practical framework of recommendations for midwives and wider healthcare staff. More than a practical set of good practice recommendations, Emma investigates a wide range of issues she believes can disproportionately and negatively affect the autistic woman's birth in comparison to her peers, such as socioeconomic factors, intersectionality, government policy and more. Emma explores the wider feminist issues around consent, autonomy and trauma for all women – autistic, disabled or otherwise. Hayley's research findings echo this, to a concerning degree, which is their motivation for writing this book and educating as many people as possible.

Hayley and Emma's shared work on the autistic birth experience

Hayley and Emma have presented at the Let's Talk Birth 2020 conference to midwives, doulas and others alongside well-known names in the birth industry including Mars Lord and Sheen Byrom, OBE. Hayley and Emma have both worked with Birthrights, an organisation that campaigns for the essential human rights of a birthing mother. Birthrights have offered to help disseminate Hayley's research findings, which offer stark reading, particularly about autonomy and informed consent.

Hayley and Emma are increasingly well known in the UK autism community, with excellent links at governmental level, to local health boards, communities and individuals. We are often the first point of call and are signposted by many well-known names as being experts on the autistic birth experience.

Karen Henry, RM, MA

Karen is a midwife, researcher and lecturer in midwifery at the University of Suffolk. She has five children and was diagnosed as autistic alongside her fourth and fifth children in 2009. Whilst training to be a midwife in 2015, Karen noticed that autistic women accessing maternity care were often unprepared for a stay in hospital, with its unfamiliar noises, smells, people and routines. She also recognised that maternity staff did not receive sufficient autism training to be able to support autistic parents.

In 2019, Karen was nominated for a Florence Nightingale Foundation scholarship and was supported to create a series of communication support plans. The idea of the plans was for women to be able to share their support needs with maternity staff in order to make care in hospitals and clinics more accessible for them. The plans were developed further in 2020 to incorporate information sharing from maternity staff so that women can be prepared and know what to expect during their pregnancy, birth and the postnatal period.

Karen completed an Autism Master of Arts at Manchester Metropolitan University in 2022 and tailored the whole programme to autistic women's experiences. This included experiences of poor mental health and being sectioned under the Mental Health Act, autistic people's experiences of employment and bullying in the workplace, the effects of hospital stays on autistic women's sensory input and the fear autistic parents experience when being referred for safeguarding and social care. Karen also extensively explored through sociological frameworks the experience of growing up as an autistic girl, how underdiagnosis and misdiagnosis commonly occurs and the reasons for this. She explored the evolution of motherhood and the values associated with 'being a good mother', then intersected this with common misconceptions associated with autistic people. Autistic women's narratives were explored in terms of the poor maternity experiences they can face; however, Karen knew that some women report excellent maternity care and so explored, through narrative enquiry, the notion that midwives with personal autism experience (either through being autistic themselves or being a mother of an autistic child) have skills, knowledge and experience that were not learnt through traditional midwifery training. From the findings, Karen was able to develop a framework for training to be co-produced and delivered by autistic women and midwives with personal autism experiences to ensure that the training for maternity staff is meaningful, relatable and memorable, and equips them with ideas to support care adjustments for autistic women. Ultimately, Karen envisages a maternity service where women feel safe and supported enough to thrive and embrace parenthood and where maternity staff feel confident to support them in this.

Introduction

Some may call it kismet that after years of living mere minutes apart, Emma and Hayley came to attend the same master's course with a focus on the same, much-overlooked topic. Upon crossing paths, we both realised that we could complement each other with our approaches to the autistic birth experience, with Hayley's MSc focusing on gathering much-needed data from autistic childbearers about their experience. At the same time, Emma created practical solutions in the form of a training package for midwives and other healthcare professionals, with complementary programmes for autistic parents or parents-to-be and their support network. Emma and Hayley have since collaborated on this topic a number of times in the past few years. Highlights have included working for Birthrights, a charity that supports human rights in childbirth, and speaking at conferences such as Let's Talk Birth and events held by the Participatory Autism Research Collective at London South Bank University. Additionally, Emma also delivered training at Community of Practice events attended by a range of professionals from across Wales, and Hayley presented her findings to the Welsh Health and Social Care Conference 2020.

Karen and Hayley's paths crossed often from 2019 onwards with their shared interest of researching the autistic birth experience. Karen's work veered into creating accessible maternity care and staff training, which subsequently led to her creating a training film for the NHS Suffolk and North East Essex Maternity Transformations project. Karen and Hayley are founding members of the Maternity Autism Research Group (MARG), whose aims are to share resources and current research for maternity staff and to support autistic women to navigate maternity care.

Karen was invited by Hayley and Emma to co-write this book because her values align with theirs. As an autistic woman and mother of an autistic daughter, Karen says:

My life is centred around my daughter who will hopefully have a baby one day. I want to contribute to education and research because when that day comes, I want her to feel embraced by maternity care that considers who she is as a person where she feels safe and supported. I will smile and think, 'I helped make that happen.'

Each and every engagement has only served to further confirm the neglect of this important topic and reinforce just how vital the need for comprehensive knowledge and guidance for both professionals and childbearers is. It is our most sincere hope that this book, grown from our experiences of pregnancy, childbirth, trauma and adjusting to parenthood, will add to the growing conversation around the autistic birth experience. This book has been built upon both experience and scientific research, engagement and professional experience, which we hope will help illustrate to professionals the specific issues autistic childbearers may encounter, and how best to support them. We also want to reassure autistic mothers and childbearers that they are not alone, that their experience is valid, recognised and even mirrored by others. Going forward, we would like to offer them help in equipping them with strategies to ensure the most positive experience of this monumental life event possible for them and their loved ones.

We have endeavoured, therefore, to make this a robust, comprehensive, yet practical and accessible guide that can not only enable understanding but also offer concrete, realistic options to make the autistic birth experience better.

NB: It's important to note that the strategies and information in this book could also be helpful for those with other conditions, such as learning disabilities, anxiety and other mental health conditions. Indeed, it is our belief that often what benefits autistic people benefits everyone.

Description of the book

This book is the stuff of dreams for the authors. While they have loved sharing their personal experiences about pregnancy, birth and motherhood, they noticed a distinct lack of scientifically approached works in this area. Hayley and Emma have both investigated a UK health board's training competency on autism and other conditions. They were surprised to learn that in order to be considered an 'autism expert midwife', only one hour of training is required. This training is not advertised as having any robust objectives, continuing practice commitments or autistic voice.

Their scientific knowledge is always the foundation from which Hayley and Emma work – whenever Hayley presents information about the autistic pain experience, this is informed by her systematic review on the subject in medical school. When Hayley presents her findings about the autistic birth experience, this is done so with the view of 250 women who answered her survey analysed appropriately and the 480 medical journals she read in and around the area of autistic transitioning and parenthood.

What the authors would like to create is a future-proof, scientifically robust book that is accessible to all those who have the ability to improve care during pregnancy, birth and aftercare for autistic women. The aim is to be able to digest chapters, one at a time, for the anxious mum/parent, and for medical professionals to read over a number of days and be able to take immediate, actionable information.

Structure of the book
Chapter 1: Background and History
This chapter will include the history of modern birth practices and how we developed to current standards, the history of autism as a diagnosis and an overview of key theories, and a 'snapshot' of present-day working knowledge.

Chapter 2: Intersectionality and Feminism
This chapter will include research and statistics on the various intersections including other co-occurring conditions and disabilities, LGBTQIA+, and other issues more common in the autistic community (e.g. domestic abuse, bullying, sexual harassment). We will also include information from ethnic minorities, including the impact of cultural differences, under-diagnosis, stigma and stereotypes, as well as the findings of reports such as the MBRRACE report. Feminism will form a foundation here, with a retrospective investigation into the roots of gender disparity in healthcare.

Chapter 3: Coexisting Conditions
This chapter will include information on commonly occurring coexisting conditions such as mental health, autoimmune, sleep and eating disorders/disordered eating and more, and their impact on pregnancy, birth and new parenthood will be discussed.

Chapter 4: Pain and Sensory Differences

The interaction between sensory systems and pain in the autistic brain will be comprehensively discussed, as well as co-occurring conditions that may make this a significant disadvantage for the autistic birth experience. This may include alexithymia, chronic pain, Ehlers–Danlos syndrome and epilepsy. Recommendations will include newly devised pain scale approaches and descriptions of behaviours that may signal interoceptive pain or sensory overwhelm.

Chapter 5: Autistic Communication

Hayley's background is linguistics and she's very interested in the practical application of Milton's 'Double Empathy Problem' in this real-world setting. Practically speaking, this will take the form of a research-based foundation about autistic communication. This will then be built upon through the lens of double empathy, including approaches and tips to help bridge this gap between communication styles.

Chapter 6: Advice for Professionals

In this chapter, we will bring together all the topics discussed in earlier chapters and consider the impact this can have on professional practice, including standards of care such as the Nursery and Midwifery Council (NMC) code. Hayley will also present findings from her original research and Emma will present her proposed training plan for healthcare professionals.

Chapter 7: Practical Strategies and Information

In this chapter, we discuss specific impacts on pregnancy, birth and parenthood for autistic people and their loved ones, and share practical advice, information and suggested strategies to improve the autistic birth experience for everyone involved.

Chapter 8: Summary and Closing Wishes

CHAPTER 1

Background and History

This chapter will include the history of modern birth practices and how we developed to current standards, the history of autism as a diagnosis and an overview of key theories, and a 'snapshot' of present-day working knowledge.

- History of autism as a concept

- Autism: key concepts

- How do these differences impact the autistic birth experience?

- Why have we overlooked the autistic birth experience?

- The autistic birth experience

- What can we do to improve the experience and outcomes of autistic women and their loved ones?

- A brief history of childbirth practice, culture and autonomy

- Current challenges in healthcare – pregnancy and birth

Autistic people have key differences in how they experience the world, in perception, processing and responses. These differences are known as 'pervasive', meaning they impact all areas of our daily life, our very being, across several domains, such as communication, interaction and sensory systems. One area of our life that they impact greatly is the experience of intimacy, relationships, pregnancy, birth and parenthood. However, this is an area that has been hugely overlooked until recent years, and exploration of the specific needs of autistic people in this area is only beginning.

This book seeks to offer information and understanding as to why the autistic birth experience is different, and how we can best support autistic people throughout the process, with specific information on how autistic differences impact each stage, insight from autistic people, and advice for healthcare professionals on what adaptations they can make to ensure the experience is as positive as it can be, because although pregnancy, birth and parenthood can be stressful, it should also be joyous – for everyone, and for too long we have failed to include neurodivergent people in this equation.

History of autism as a concept

'Autism' is a word you will probably have heard more frequently in recent years. With a growing understanding of the condition, how it can vary in presentation and increasing clinical expertise in this area, more people are being diagnosed with autism than ever before. However, autism is not a new phenomenon, with the word itself first being used in 1908, and scientists and academics speculating on accounts of autism in literature much further back still. Although we may not always have seen and recognised autism as we are beginning to, it has always existed as a rich strand in the tapestry of humanity.

Our first leap forward in the study of autism and developing clinical criteria occurred in 1942 when two Austrian psychiatrists, Leo Kanner and Hans Asperger, first began to mould our understanding of autism (Fletcher-Watson & Happé 2019).

Leo Kanner was considered the world's first child psychiatrist. In 1930, he moved to Johns Hopkins University Hospital in Baltimore, USA, where he worked on the first profile of autism. Kanner was perceived by some as a controversial figure in the history of autism, working with Bruno Bettelheim who was an early proponent of applied behaviour analysis (ABA), using behavioural modification in an attempt to control autistic characteristics, and even using methods such as electric shock treatment to provide negative reinforcement for those displaying autistic traits. Bettelheim and Kanner also suggested that autism was related to 'refrigerator mothers' – mothers who lacked maternal nurturing and were cold and detached – causing the stigma around autism to increase and leading to misunderstanding and unwarranted concern over parenting ability (Bettelheim & Kanner in Fletcher-Watson & Happé 2019).

Hans Asperger, who carried out his work in a clinic in Vienna, developed the profile of autism that came to be known as Asperger's syndrome. For many years, he was viewed as a positive figure by the autistic community, due to his positive focus on the strengths that autistic characteristics may provide, even stating that 'for success in science or art, a dash of autism is necessary' (Silberman 2016). He seemed fond of the children he worked with, working on their academic development in the mornings and encouraging them to pursue passions in music, arts, etc. in the afternoons. Indeed, some of the children Hans Asperger worked with at his clinic went on to excel, with one going on to win a Nobel prize and another finding a flaw in Isaac Newton's work. Not all was as it seemed, however; many autistic people were dismayed at the toppling of this seemingly paternal figure when it was discovered that Asperger was an active member of the Nazi Party, playing an important role in eugenics by sending children to death camps, facts he later distorted by altering records of his work.

Decades later, the first genetic links in autism were seemingly confirmed during work by Michael Rutter and his colleagues, which focused on monozygotic (identical) and dizygotic (non-identical) twins (Tick *et al.* 2016). Where the twins were identical, meaning both formed from one egg that split, the instance of both being autistic was statistically significant, suggesting there are clear genetic factors that lead to a person being autistic. To this day, the exact genetic factors remain largely unknown, and autism is believed to be a complex mix of genetic, environmental, neurological and immunological factors.

Norwegian-American clinical psychologist Ole Ivor Lovaas, based at the University of California, Los Angeles (UCLA), pioneered a form of ABA known as the Lovaas Method. The focus here was on improving language and interpersonal communication skills for autistic people. While many families have reported their autistic family member's behaviour benefitted from ABA, there is widespread condemnation of this approach from the adult autistic community. Those who have experienced such interventions have reported psychological distress, from low self-esteem and identity issues to complex post-traumatic stress disorder. In addition to these community reports, many modern autism research academics have carried out systematic literature searches to evaluate the effectiveness of such approaches. Research by Fletcher-Watson *et al.* (2014) suggests that after teaching 'Theory of Mind' based skills (e.g. emotion recognition, social communication) to autistic people there was 'little evidence of maintenance of that skill, generalisation to other settings, or developmental effects on related skills'. Many other scholars have reported that similar evaluations of early intensive behavioral interventions (including the Lovaas Method and ABA, including 'Theory of Mind' skills) have shown not only ineffectiveness of such interventions but active harm being done to the identity of the autistic persons subjected to interventions (Shkedy, Shkedy & Sandoval-Norton 2021).

Our current understanding of autism is still informed strongly by the seminal work of Lorna Wing (1981a) and Judith Gould, two scientists who were instrumental in the National Autistic Society (NAS), viewed as the most prominent charity devoted to autism in the UK to this day. Wing and Gould were the first to present the idea of autism as a spectrum condition, presenting the idea of the 'triad of impairments', a concept that suggests autistic people have key differences in social communication, social interaction and social imagination, which influences both our understanding of autism and the diagnostic tools and criteria we rely upon still.

In recent years, there has been what some may refer to as an autistic culture shift, with many autistic people giving first-person accounts of how it feels to be autistic, relating their perceptions of the world. This has influenced policy, services and research, with more focus being given to collaborative research that involves autistic people more wholly in the process, rather than conclusions being drawn from study and observation of autistic people alone. Also, autistic people are shaping the narrative more and more, fighting for policy and services that truly meet their needs, and working to ensure the autistic voice is not only heard but listened to. This has unfortunately caused some conflict in the autistic community, particularly between some parents of autistic children and autistic people, but politically autism has been very much on the agenda, with Wales, Scotland and Northern Ireland having autism policies, and England establishing the Autism Act in 2009. Media portrayals of autism have also become more varied, showing a more diverse range of autistic people, which is a positive step forward in increasing understanding and refuting misconceptions and stereotypes in society.

Pioneered in the UK by Uta Frith – a mentor to Simon Baron-Cohen, whose name is now almost synonymous with autism – 'autism awareness' was becoming more widespread by the 1960s. This was further expanded by Lorna Wing and Judith Gould, whose 'triad of impairments' – mentioned above – still underpin many of the diagnostic tools used today. The year 1985 saw Baron-Cohen's seminal collection of essays, *Theory of Mind*, in which he linked observations of autistic deficits in false belief and mind-reading tasks to theories about a lack of empathy (Baron-Cohen, Leslie & Frith 1985). The triad of impairments and Theory of Mind continue to influence diagnostic tools, as well as support and research centred around the autistic population.

Contemporaneous to Baron-Cohen's *Theory of Mind* in the UK, the Australian sociologist Judith Singer (2017) developed her theory of 'neurodiversity', a portmanteau coined from 'neurological' and 'diversity'. Singer used the term to represent her ideology, a movement based on an acceptance of all varieties of 'neurotypes' present in society as natural and intrinsic to the human race.

More positive progress has been achieved due to the work of Singer, which focused on difference rather than deficit, with neurodivergent conditions such as attention deficit hyperactivity disorder (ADHD), dyslexia, dyspraxia and dyscalculia also falling under this umbrella (Singer 2017). We are seeing a rise in the amount of work by autistic academics and researchers, such as that of Damian Milton, whose Double Empathy Theory also challenged perceptions and beliefs of autism (Milton 2012).

Autistic people are also coming together, both in real terms and via social media, not only to accept but to celebrate their autistic identity, with self-advocacy being promoted and supported and the creation of autistic pride events across the UK. Social media has also provided an accessible platform for many autistic people to blog and vlog about their experiences and feelings and connect with the wider autistic community. This has positive impacts not only in shifting the perceptions of autism in society but also in protecting the self-esteem of autistic people, as they find a place where they can fit and be accepted, understood and celebrated for who they are rather than feeling shame and guilt as many did due to deficit-based models of autism and stigma in the community. Work by Monique Botha showed that this community support was vital in protecting mental health and reducing self-harm and suicidality in the autistic community (Botha & Frost 2020). On a wider perspective, one could argue such issues result from an interaction of both models of disability – medical professionals' view of autism and 'deficits' and the view of societal norms and disabling environments.

Research focus – cure narrative or support narrative?

Considering the context of the ever-evolving narrative landscape surrounding autism and autistic communities, the orientation of research is increasingly answering community calls to adopt the social model of disability and identity-first language (as opposed to person-first language – e.g. 'person with autism'). However, medical models in certain aspects of healthcare prevail, as well as affecting the narratives in the public sphere and media.

Reducing autistic lives, experiences and identities to a reductive symbol or small set of stereotyped behaviours does little to improve awareness; this is particularly true for autistic people who are not cisgender white males.

Organisations are slowly adapting their approach to embrace the changes called for by the autistic community, but such changes are by no means being effected at a uniform and reliable pace.

A promotion for the NYU Child Study Center in the United States used a 'ransom note' design, portraying autism as a kidnapper. In another campaign for the UK charity Action for Children, autism was depicted as a child-enveloping monster that had to be destroyed to allow a boy to live a normal life. A third presentation, the film 'I Am Autism' distributed by US-based charity Autism Speaks, married narration in the style of a horror-film trailer with scenes from the lives of stressed families affected by autism (Waltz 2017).

Even from a fundamentally linguistic perspective, the way autism is referred to in such spheres directly relates to how this community is perceived and therefore treated in real-world situations. The influential Saussurean model of the relationship between signifier and *signified* enables us to appreciate the mutually inclusive nature of how we talk about concepts. For example, autistic people or autism as the *signified* is directly shaped and informed by the *signifiers* used by the majority of the population – that is, the predominant neurotype or general population without autism.

As Stuart Hall (1997) has noted, it is through signs and symbols that concepts and ideas are represented, and within these representations via language that cultural meanings are produced. This can be observed in representations purveyed by disability charities, which function to construct a medical model of disability and place themselves in a role of care, cure and control in relation to it (Waltz 2017).

It's worth considering how such symbols, images, stereotypes and other representations of the autistic population subliminally inform the expectations we have of autistic people. From a fundamental perspective, changing the *signifiers* is more than a PR exercise, and rather a monumental but essential task in improving autism acceptance throughout the lifespan.

Autistic voices

We have also begun what some term an 'autistic culture shift'. With the advent of the neurodiversity movement (Singer 1999), likened in some ways to the gay rights movement, autistic and neurodiverse people are becoming more empowered and connected and collectively have a stronger voice – 'Nothing about us without us' (Loomes 2018; Milton *et al.* 2019). This has meant many more autistic advocates, activists and participants in research and co-production of services and resources, truly beginning a shift in the narrative and drawing attention to issues previously overlooked, including autistic birth (Hoekstra *et al.* 2018).

Autism: key concepts

This section will include a brief overview of key concepts related to autism, including:

- social communication and interaction

- social imagination

- Theory of Mind

- sensory differences

- executive functioning (monotropism, tendril theory)

- central coherence

- emotional regulation.

Social communication and interaction, sensory issues and pain will be covered in depth in subsequent chapters, but a brief introduction is given here.

Social communication and interaction

Autistic people have key differences in the way they communicate and interact. These form two of the three parts of the triad – a concept by Lorna Wing and Judith Gould that informs our diagnostic criteria.

This can mean:

- they are non- or minimally verbal

- they can be misunderstood

- they struggle with the complexities of social interaction

- they find being around others difficult

- they struggle to make or maintain friendships

- they place value on different methods of communication.

Social imagination

Social imagination forms the third part of the 'triad'.

In essence, it means imagining:

- how others may be thinking and feeling

- what might happen next

- the consequence of our actions – and sometimes a lack of age-appropriate awareness of danger

- how our actions could impact others' responses.

Difficulty with social imagination can contribute greatly to the world feeling like a very confusing and uncertain place for autistic people to navigate, leading them to rely heavily on routines and struggle with change and transitions as a result. This not only relates to major changes such as moving home, relationship changes or changing schools or jobs, but also in moving from one activity to the next on a daily basis.

Autistic people also often develop intense interests, subjects or topics which they hyperfocus on and can learn a great deal about. This can be a strength in the joy and comfort these interests provide and also lead to success when channelled into studies and career development. However, this 'hyperfocus' can sometimes cause difficulties when socialising with others (e.g. not understanding others' lack of interest in certain topics or misreading the social appropriateness of the topic they would like to share information about). For instance, while it is well known that autistic people often build rapport by sharing information or facts, this isn't necessarily the case for the general population, who more often gauge such matters through small talk and other phatic communication. (Phatic communication refers to aspects of language that exist purely to pass time or build rapport.)

This can be illustrated by the hypothetical example of a young autistic woman who tried to engage in what she thought was small talk with a stranger at a bus stop. Her attempt saw her generously sharing facts about her special interest, serial killers, without taking into account the stranger's perception of her motivation for sharing this information on a dark winter's night at a bus stop. In line with our 'double empathy' approach in this book (Milton 2017), we will view this exchange as a *mismatch of salience* in the specific context as opposed to viewing the autistic person's input as merely wrong or a deficit of typical small talk. There is inherently a discordance between communication styles, which can have immediate and critical effects on the resulting unintended consequences.

Social imagination differences often get confused with imagination linked to creativity, but this is a myth; it refers to *social* imagination only – many autistic people are very creative.

Other observable differences may present the autistic individual with difficulty picking up non-verbal clues about how others are feeling. Considering how integral these normally unconscious skills are to success in everyday life in the neurotypically designed world, it's not difficult to imagine the vast number of unintended consequences that may result from this difference. Many neurotypical people can recall a time when similar misunderstandings have occurred to them; with reflection, this can lead to a degree of empathy for the difficulties autistic people will inherently face. However, the magnitude of the effects of this issue surpass personal and interpersonal levels: mismatches of social communication styles can lead to inaccessibility on policy, legal and societal levels.

Theory of mind

As briefly discussed earlier in this book, intrinsic to these social imagination differences is the concept of 'Theory of Mind', a term used by Sir Simon Baron-Cohen in his seminal works from the 1980s (Baron-Cohen *et al.* 1985). It refers to the difficulty autistic individuals may have in 'putting themselves in someone else's shoes'. Moreover, it is described as a difficulty/inability to see things from someone else's perspective, or to understand that another's 'inner world' (thoughts, beliefs or interests) may differ from your own. This autism characteristic may also make it difficult to anticipate how others may behave or feel. In a healthcare context, this may mean questions are not answered in the manner expected and the ability to self-advocate or provide informed consent is diminished or absent.

Many scholars believe Theory of Mind can continue to develop over the lifespan – that is, development is asynchronous and atypical but not necessarily absent – and it can be developed with intervention such as skills training. However, as previously noted, the applicability of the training has been questioned and the autistic community voice on the matter has long spoken out against these interventions.

Additionally, on a human and interpersonal level, it is worth stating that autistic people can be empathetic. Regardless of diagnosis, our personalities, experiences and defining qualities are as varied and complex as any other population. While the typical behaviours, language or other symbolic gestures of empathy may be different in the autistic individual, the true innate sensation of empathy cannot be discounted. Many autistic people report being hyper-empathetic to the needs of others, some reporting that the social context of their response or behaviour to this is different or difficult to initiate for different reasons. There is an argument that the highly driven need to gauge and respond correctly to the needs of others is a trauma response – a protective mechanism learned by the autistic individual to provide themselves with the best chances of survival, whether in a social context or a practical everyday sense. Overall, the authors of this book suggest that the perception and demonstration of empathy in autistic people may differ but not be lesser than that of the neurotypical person, and that adequate respect/regard should be given to this in all contexts.

Women are responsible for child rearing responsibility because of the unequal distribution of labour in the household (Criado-Perez 2019; Oakley 1974, 1979). Almost from birth, girls are considered within the context of motherhood and their ability to attach and bond with a child as mothers, yet autistic women report being perceived as incapable of mothering qualities. Much of the information available for health professionals is based upon highly criticised psychological studies which claim autistic people, amongst other deficits, are unable to empathise (Baron-Cohen 2003, 2006, 2009). Such studies are based on male childhood presentations of autism, which are not representative of the experiences autistic women who report motherhood to be 'the most stable relationship they have ever had' (Burton 2016). In fact, many autistic mothers speak about putting their child's needs above their own, which certainly demonstrates empathy and seeing things from another's point of view (Hill 2017).

Sensory differences

What we see, hear, feel, smell and taste gives us information about our environment and ourselves. Our sensory systems work together to help us make sense of the world and how to act within it. Our bodies and the environment send our brains information through the senses that we process and organise to understand the world and respond appropriately.

Autistic people often have key differences in sensory perception, processing and responses.

This can mean they are under- or over-sensitive to sensory information, or a complex mix of both.

It can affect all eight senses:

- sight: visual

- sound: auditory

- smell: olfactory

- taste: gustatory

- touch: tactile

- balance: vestibular

- spatial awareness: proprioception

- interoception: 'the eighth sense'.

These sensory differences and related conditions will be explored further in Chapter 4.

Executive functioning

Executive functioning describes the cognitive processes that enable us to think, plan, organise and generally carry out the activities required in daily life. Many autistic individuals will struggle with executive functioning. Temple Grandin, for example, famously described her inability to hold one piece of information in her mind while manipulating the next step in the sequence.

Our brains comprise two systems: automatic and executive. It is estimated that on a daily basis we use our automatic system 80–90% of the time and the executive system 10–20% of the time. The executive system requires purposeful regulatory effort – frequent mental pauses and ceaseless self-regulation, which can prove exhausting.

Executive functioning happens in the frontal lobe and describes the processes in the brain that allow us to think, plan, prioritise, organise. It is the brain's ability to receive, process, hold on to and work with information. It allows us to filter distractions and switch gears.

It encompasses a set of skills including three types of brain function – working memory, mental flexibility and self-control – affecting skills and functions such as:

- **Planning:** Making plans, carrying them out, setting and reaching goals.

- **Focus:** Concentrating on important things, whilst filtering out less important distractions.

- **Impulse control:** Regulating our emotions, internal state and reactions.

- **Awareness:** Being aware of our environment and the people in it, as well as our role in the situation.

- **Flexibility:** Being able to adapt to change, 'switch gears' and cope with interruptions.

- **Reflection:** Being able to reflect on experiences and situations, and gather and use the information to grow and learn, as well as being able to evaluate how we are doing. Difficulty reflecting may mean surprise at negative feedback.

- **Attention and focus:** Being able to focus on a person or task for a time and shifting that attention when needed (switching gears). There are lots of ideas/theories about how this is impacted in neurodivergent people, including monotropism,[1] intense interests and tendril theory.[2]

- **Perseverance:** The ability to stick with a task and not give up, even when it becomes challenging.

- **Time management:** Having an accurate understanding of how long tasks will take and using time wisely and effectively to accomplish them.

- **Organisation:** Keeping track of things physically and mentally.

People are not born with executive functioning skills, just the potential to develop them. For people with a different developmental trajectory, executive function may also develop differently. This explains why people who are neurodivergent, autistic, ADHD, etc. may struggle with executive function. Executive function skills continue to develop over time, with the full range of abilities continuing to grow and mature throughout childhood, adolescence and early adulthood. These skills may develop in a different order and at a different rate for people with neurodevelopmental differences.

It can be useful to think of our executive functioning abilities as the brain's air traffic control system or command centre. For example, it is like an airport having the effective ability to manage multiple arrivals and departures across a complicated network of runways.

---

1   Monotropism describes the tendency to focus attention on one thing at a time; the person will sometimes miss things outside this tunnel of attention which might have aided understanding.
2   Tendril theory suggests that when focusing on a task, neurodivergent people send out 'tendrils of thought' which expand and branch out; when asked to suddenly switch focus or move from one task to another, all of the tendrils get 'ripped out'. The theory suggests that the person needs time to file away all of these tendrils before they can focus on a new task.

Working memory, which may be thought of as the brain's GPS, describes the mental processes that allow us to hold information in our minds while working with it. The stronger your working memory, the less work your brain must undertake for tasks (like a computer's processing power). Like a GPS booting up for a new voyage, the brain begins a new task by referring to its maps – sensory images logged and stored in non-verbal working memory – and the verbal commands and inner voice images help act and voice guides. The purposes of executive functional skills and the impact of difficulties with executive function are summarised in Table 1.1.

Table 1.1 Executive functioning skills: purposes and impacts

Skill	What it means	Impact
Working memory	Helps keep key information in mind	Trouble remembering directions (even if the person has taken notes or the instructions have been repeated several times)
Impulse control	Helps to keep their own feelings regulated Helps to think before acting	Prone to overreact May struggle with criticism and regrouping when something goes wrong May blurt out inappropriate things May have little/no sense of danger
Mental/cognitive flexibility	Allows you to adjust to the unexpected	Struggles to cope when things change suddenly/unexpectedly Frustration when asked to look at things from another perspective
Task initiation and motivation	Task initiation is the ability to independently take action and start tasks when needed It is the process that allows you to just begin something even when you don't really want to	Inertia/motivation difficulties can mean a person may freeze up, not know where to begin or be unable to take the first steps

Neuroplasticity

The neuroplasticity that enables us to continue learning and evolving throughout our lives has pros and cons:

- **Positive:** We can continue to build and improve executive function across the lifespan.

- **Negative:** These skills and processes are subject to disruption from external influences across the lifespan.

It is important to note that not only are the person's existing executive function skills impacted, but also the ability to embed new executive function skills can be affected, particularly when a person is in a state of anxiety or stress, as is often the case for autistic people.

> Imagine how many steps there are in making a cup of tea or a piece of toast. Most people with good executive function/working memory will hold the steps in their head easily and complete many of them on 'autopilot'. As such, many neurotypical people who attend my executive function training often respond with between six and ten steps for these tasks. In reality, the steps are far greater – the record we have had written in a training activity was 70 but the attendee could have kept writing! A standard response may include a step such as 'boil the kettle', but there are myriad smaller components to bringing this to fruition which I won't bore you with here. For an autistic/neurodivergent person who struggles with working memory, these 'simple' tasks can feel overwhelming or impossible. Worse still, when we somehow muddle through and make that cup of tea, our loved ones are often not impressed by the important step we managed to forget along the way – such as putting the milk back in the fridge and unintentionally causing it to spoil. There are days when I struggle so much with everyday tasks that it feels like 'trying to nail jelly to a wall'. For years I believed I was lazy, useless or not trying hard enough. People couldn't understand how I could be academically capable but struggled with simple everyday tasks. I couldn't understand it. Coming to learn about executive functioning made sense of so much of my life and helped me to understand myself more. I try not to internally berate myself as much – work in progress, though! Executive functioning virtually disappeared after my child's birth and I remember looking at the bottle steriliser and just crying – the thought of trying to complete a new task was completely overwhelming.
>
> *Emma*

Difficulties with executive function are sometimes referred to as executive dysfunction. These present similarly to the phenomenon often referred to as cognitive fog, or 'cog-fog', which often impacts people with conditions that affect their energy levels. These can include:

- time blindness – difficulties understanding and managing time

- procrastination

- working memory

- self-regulation – sudden emotional changes

- organisation

- decision making

- managing belongings – being prone to misplacing/losing items

- forgetfulness

- distraction and concentration difficulties.

It is imperative that executive dysfunction does not get misinterpreted as bad behaviour; unfortunately, difficulties in controlling impulses, focusing attention, staying organised and following instructions can sometimes be viewed as rudeness, laziness or a 'bad attitude'. This perception can lead to a lack of support, unhelpful punitive measures and low self-esteem.

It is also important to remember that executive functioning ability is not static: it fluctuates with stress, anxiety and other external factors. For neurodivergent people, the ability to hyperfocus on certain tasks or activities whilst struggling to engage with others can look like purposeful selective attention, compounding the potential perception of bad behaviour.

Executive functioning difficulties can have a widespread impact on our lives, making everyday tasks difficult and causing feelings of guilt and shame which can impact self-esteem and overall mental wellbeing.

Phrases that might be familiar to people who struggle with executive functioning may include:

- 'How can you be so intelligent but have no common sense?'

- 'Why can't you just apply yourself?'

- 'It's just a simple task for heaven's sake!'

The stigma faced from others and internalised within ourselves can be devastating, increasing our feelings of overwhelm and compounding existing difficulties with this additional mental/emotional load.

Central coherence

First described by Uta Frith in 1989, who theorised that autistic individuals have 'weak central coherence', the concept is often described as the ability to 'see the bigger picture'. Autistic people are often far better at focusing on the details and can find it really difficult to form these into a cohesive whole and put them into context. This may be best described as an inherent hyperfocus consequence of the well-known phrase 'can't see the wood for trees' – except that it's not something that can be easily changed with a shift in perspective but is an inherent difference in neurological wiring.

A good analogy to understand this concept is that of shining a torch against a wall. The closer you move the torch to the wall, the brighter but narrower the beam of the light; as you move the torch further away, the beam widens but also dims. It could be suggested that autistic people are just closer to the wall with their torches – which can be both a strength and a challenge in differing ways.

Applying context to any of these characteristics is essential for explanation, understanding and appreciation of unintended consequences. What is often described as a quirky, stereotypical personality trait with embarrassing social consequences can be a very real 'blessing and a curse' dichotomy for autistic people. Using the example of a new parent, noticing changes in a baby's wellbeing that others may not notice can be a genuinely life-saving skill, or it could be perceived as obsessive symptom-spotting and suspected as a case of fabricated or induced illness (FII – formerly known as Munchausen's by proxy). (If you'd like to learn more about FII and the autistic community, please do look up the work of Shona Murphy on Twitter or via Sheffield Hallam University.)

Emotional regulation

Autistic people can often have trouble managing or even identifying their emotions.

It can mean we react strongly to rejection, change moods quickly and are very sensitive to the emotions of those around us. This can sometimes result in extreme, unpredictable or unwise/inappropriate behaviour.

Emotional regulation is often affected in the commonly coexisting condition of ADHD. Individuals with ADHD may also experience rejection sensitivity dysphoria (RSD), which means that a person with this condition experiences extreme emotional pain in response to implied criticism, rejection or perceived failure. While these experiences may be uncomfortable for anyone to experience, for those with RSD the emotional reaction and pain can reach unbearable levels, to the extent that it can mimic the symptoms of mood disorders and trigger self-harming behaviours or suicidal ideation.

Likewise, autistic people may also strive for perfection and aim to avoid rejection or criticism. Despite some of the historical myths around autistic people having a 'lack of empathy', many autistic people report an excess of empathy, or being 'hyper-empathetic', feeling others' emotions as strongly as their own. The difference for autistic people often lies in the distinction between cognitive and affective empathy, and while we may not consciously pick up subtleties of how others are feeling and why, we are often attuned in another sense, or we may need more information to understand and empathise dependent on the situation and the individual.

> It feels like being a 'raw nerve' in the world, like I'm a sponge that absorbs the emotions of those around me. Not just loved ones, but the perception of pain, shame or other emotions experienced by people individually or collectively around the world can overwhelm me, to the point that I have to 'detach' and 'hibernate' to protect myself. I remember reading about the German word *Weltschmerz*, which roughly translated means 'world sadness', and it resonated with me hugely. I loved history at school, but found it overwhelming, both *because* I could almost walk into the emotions of the people described and *in spite of it*.
>
> *Emma*

Autistic meltdown, shutdown and burnout, and the fight, flight or freeze response

A meltdown occurs when a person loses control for a period of time, possibly resulting in damage to property, self or others. This damage to self and others may be physical or verbal. A shutdown can occur for the same reasons, but the effects are often much more internal. Shutdowns can be missed/more difficult to identify than meltdowns, as often the person will seem to be withdrawn, distracted and/or not communicative.

Shutdown and meltdown can be seen as an expression of the fight, flight or freeze response.

During this response, there is a redirection from essential skills as we switch from executive to automatic response circuits. This means a reduction/loss of executive function, overloading the ability to use these skills, such as verbal communication or decision making, or to learn and embed new skills or process information.

Both mean a crisis point has been reached but they look very different:

Meltdown	Shutdown
Display extreme behaviour such as: • self-harm • shouting • aggression – kicking, hitting, biting	Complete withdrawal: • non-responsive to communication • cease to interact with world • retreat to 'safe space'/hide • lie down where they are • unable to move
EXTERNAL	INTERNAL

A meltdown or shutdown often has three stages:

- rumbling phase
- active meltdown/shutdown
- recovery phase.

It is vital to remember that meltdowns are not tantrums; they do not happen as a means to exert control but rather because of a loss of control. During meltdown or shutdown, the person has often lost many functional abilities, decision making, communication and even motor control, and they are often ashamed, remorseful and exhausted after a meltdown or shutdown. Sometimes meltdown or shutdown can seem unpredictable and sudden, but with time we can learn to recognise signs of the 'rumbling' phase. It takes time and effort to identify 'triggers'.

When an autistic person pushes through overload for an extended period of time, experiencing more regular shutdowns and meltdowns, they may enter a phase referred to as autistic burnout, which could be described as an 'extended shutdown'. In burnout, we are likely to experience high levels of fatigue, more difficulties with concentration and communication, and even more sensory sensitivities and physical pain. It can reduce our functioning substantially for days, weeks, months or even years. This is why it is so key to avoid reaching overload wherever possible and to introduce pacing and management strategies to enable autistic people to manage their energy levels and social battery (the amount of energy a person has for socialising). Strategies to help with this are detailed in Chapter 7.

The following description of shutdown and burnout is from a previously published blog by Emma (Durman 2023):

> I often say that autistic shutdown is a bit like disk defragmentation. Do you remember that maintenance tool computers had? It showed all the

information and code that was mixed up, stored securely and safely but not organised properly.

It displayed on the screen as lots and lots of tiny coloured boxes. I used to love watching it run, all the boxes slowly grouping and categorising into familiar categories of blue, red and green. What was a mish-mash of primary colour would become a neat set of colours. It brought me a deep sense of joy and calm to think of all the organisation happening in the system.

Autistic shutdown, or even just that enhanced recovery time we need after socialising or other activities, always makes me think of this. It's like I've taken in all this information, a myriad of chaotic colours that need to be sorted, made sense of. I'm pretty good at retaining information, but sometimes accessing that information takes an immense amount of work – especially if I've been 'ignoring my maintenance'. We've all done it – metaphorically clicked the 'remind me in 24 hours' button over and over again. When I push through and 'store up' these essential maintenance tasks, the more bogged down, sluggish and prone to error my system becomes. If you have to sort through piles of paperwork to find one piece of information, that's a lot harder than opening a filing cabinet and navigating to the relevant file!

If I don't carry out my defragmentation regularly – i.e. spend the time processing, replaying, making sense of and organising all that information I've collected – eventually my system will start to crash. I won't be able to run essential programs, I might lose data, and eventually even getting my operating system to switch on and respond will become near impossible. That's autistic burnout – when you enter a shutdown so long and huge it becomes impossible to function for an extended length of time. It's a very scary place to be in, because all the data is in there rattling around, and the world keeps 'pressing the keys' trying to get a response, but you can't successfully process it in or out. It's like being lost in a sea of multicoloured boxes so vast and overwhelming you feel you may never sort them out.

Self-care is necessary and vital for everyone. But things can reach critical levels faster and more catastrophically for autistic people. Our emotional regulation and executive functioning often look very different from that of non-autistic/neurotypical people, so our self-care becomes an even more essential part of life, often for longer periods. We are often feeling and processing and experiencing so much so differently, and in environments designed for the predominant neurotype, not ours.

So bear in mind when an autistic person needs more downtime, more self-care, and can engage in fewer social or other activities than you might expect, that these aren't acts of luxury or indulgence or 'special treatment'. We are ensuring we have all the time we need to sort our little coloured boxes, so we can run properly, efficiently. Given this time and understanding, we can have the best possible outcomes for ourselves, our community and society.

Demand-avoidant profiles, extreme demand avoidance (EDA)/pathological demand avoidance (PDA)

A demand-avoidant profile, sometimes referred to as pathological demand avoidance (PDA), or more recently as extreme demand avoidance (EDA), is said to be a complex profile of autism that presents differently with distinct challenges.

Many people who report having demand-avoidant profiles also claim to face additional difficulties in diagnosis and support, have problems in education and may exhibit more difficult behaviours.

Demand-avoidant profiles are not currently recognised in the diagnostic manuals, and understanding and tailored support is scarce.

Criteria for demand avoidance were published by Elizabeth Newson (Newson, Le Maréchal & David 2003), setting out eight potential characteristics.

1. Extreme avoidance of demands

The most important characteristic in the criteria, present in 100% of cases, is an extreme, pervasive resistance/avoidance of everyday demands.

This even relates to demands the individual places upon themselves and demands that are things they would very much like to do.

Individuals will often employ a wide variety of avoidant behaviours which range from aggressive to seemingly skilled socially strategic, including:

- diverting attention
  - steering conversation
  - delaying tactics
  - 'Yes, but later'
- excuses
  - 'I'm poorly'

- – 'I'm busy'
- – pretending to be unable to do something
- refusal
  - – refusing flatly
  - – disruptive behaviour
  - – aggression
- parrying
  - – 'Come look in my mirror' – 'But I have my own mirror'
  - – disengagement
  - – sensible reasons why
  - – humour.

2. Passive early history

Newson found that a high proportion of those with EDA were described by their caregivers as passive or placid in the first year of their life – for example, nearly half did not reach for their toys or dropped them when they were offered. She noted that the child only became more 'actively resistant' when more was expected of them (e.g. when starting nursery). Parents had often made quite significant accommodations without realising the issues until external demands were placed upon the child – what Newson referred to as 'velvet gloves'.

3. Comfortable in role play

Individuals with a demand-avoidant profile are often extremely comfortable in role play and pretence, sometimes to an extreme extent, where the lines between reality and pretence can become blurred. They are also likely to role-play a persona of an authority figure, a role that often requires them to oversee and direct others. They may also use role play as a strategy to avoid demands, and it seems that this withdrawal into fantasy may also be a form of self-protection.

4. Surface sociability

People with demand-avoidant profiles are often very 'people-oriented' and may have learnt many social niceties. They will often use charm in their repertoire of avoidance strategies and can seem exceptionally well tuned into what might prove an effective strategy with particular people. However, this sociability appears to be 'skin deep' and can be very misleading, with the individual actually being socially naive in many ways beneath the surface, with a lack of depth to their understanding of the social world. This can lead to overly domineering responses.

5. Lability of mood

People with demand-avoidant profiles have been reported to characteristically switch from one mood to another very suddenly (e.g. from happy and content to distraught). This has been described by some as a 'switch going on and off' or 'Jekyll and Hyde'. For example, hugging may become strangling, kisses may turn to bites. These emotional changes can seem very dramatic and unpredictable, and while at first glance this can be likened to the emotional regulation difficulties experienced in general autism profiles, the difference is often in the switch back from overwhelmed, angry or distraught to happy, content and enthusiastic.

> 'He can go from 0 to 90 faster than any car in existence – and from 90 to 0 at the same rate.'
>
> 'You are always walking on eggshells.'

6. Obsessive behaviour

Strong fascinations and intense interests are common in autistic people – so this criterion alone does not distinguish demand-avoidant profiles from classic presentations. However, the subjects of fixations for those with PDA tend to be social in nature and often revolve around specific individuals.

7. Possible neurological involvement

Newson noted what she referred to as possible neurological involvement, such as:

- absences
- tics
- floppy in infancy
- delay in meeting motor milestones

- clumsiness.

Although this aspect remains under-researched, it seems this may be linked to the early passivity described in the profile as well as to avoidance. For example, passivity may mean less motivation to talk, crawl, walk, while absences may be neurological or they may be a form of disengagement.

8. Language

Some early language delay is common; this seems to be dependent on their overall intellectual ability and part of their early passivity, and there is often an accelerated 'striking and sudden' degree of catch-up. There seems to be less difficulty generally with eye contact/non-verbal cues and pragmatics of language, though there is often still a mismatch between expressive and receptive language which likely links to surface sociability.

Research suggests that, much like other autistic profiles, EDA is very much rooted in anxiety. In fact, it is suggested that demand avoidant profiles are best understood as an anxiety-driven need for control.

> PDA is best understood as an anxiety-driven need to be in control and avoid other people's demands and expectations.
>
> *Christie*

Anxiety and excitement sit close to each other on the spectrum of emotions so each can overlap and have the same effect.

Intolerance of uncertainty

Newcastle University conducted research which found that intolerance of uncertainty (IU) and anxiety were both associated with PDA behaviour in children, and that IU was even more strongly associated with PDA than anxiety.

They found PDA behaviour can be understood as an expression of IU and anxiety in this possible hierarchy of responses:

- uncertain situation

- attempt to control aspects of the situation to reduce uncertainty

- withdrawing to fantasy or mentally disengaging (avoidance)

- loss of control over emotions and behaviour meltdown.

Identifying EDA

EDA doesn't appear in either of the diagnostic manuals – the *Diagnostic and Statistical Manual of Mental Disorders* (DSM-V) (American Psychiatric Association (APA) 2013) or the International Statistical Classification of Diseases (ICD-10) (World Health Organization (WHO) 2019). However, clinicians are increasingly diagnosing with terminology such as 'autism with a demand-avoidant profile' or 'autism and oppositional defiant disorder (ODD)/conduct disorder (CD)'. In some areas, it can be seemingly impossible to get a diagnosis of EDA. It is down to clinician discretion. Perhaps the biggest difficulty is that some of the characteristics of EDA seem to 'exclude' an autism diagnosis – which leads to no diagnosis and support in some cases. A PDA Society survey (2016) found half of diagnostic professionals would identify PDA, while research by Gore-Langton and Fredrickson (2015, 2016) found this division over recognition compounded delays faced by the autistic community in accessing diagnosis and support, with families feeling increasingly isolated and misunderstood. Research and guidance remain sparse (small-scale studies which may show confirmation bias), although it highlights the crisis faced by individuals with this profile and their close supporters.

It is vitally important to recognise that behaviours resulting from demand avoidance reflect an inability rather than being purposely difficult.

> Those with EDA can be labelled as naughty, defiant or even psychotic as it can be extremely hard for staff to recognise and accept that violent, shocking and strategic behaviours are forms of panic attacks, needing reassurance rather than reprimand. (Eaton & Banting 2012)

There have been tools developed in recent years which may aid clinicians in identifying demand-avoidant profiles, although they are not classed as diagnostic. These include:

- EDA-Q (Extreme Demand Avoidance Questionnaire) (O'Nions *et al.* 2013)

- DISCO Subset (a subset of questions from the larger DISCO (Diagnostic Interview for Social and Communication Disorders) which have been researched for effectiveness in identifying EDA characteristics)

- Coventry Grid (a tool used initially to help clinicians distinguish autism and attachment disorder which has been modified to help clinicians distinguish demand-avoidant profiles)

- EDAQ-A (Extreme Demand Avoidance Questionnaire – Adult), a modification of O'Nions *et al.*'s original questionnaire for adults by Vincent Egan and colleagues (Egan, Linenberg & O'Nions 2019).

Do we need EDA?

There is still debate around whether EDA as a classification is needed or if it is covered by autism and coexisting conditions like ODD, personality disorders, conduct disorder, etc. However, it seems these diagnoses fall short in some ways of the full criteria of EDA, leaving individuals, parents/carers and professionals in a difficult position where they do not feel that the diagnosis truly fits their profile of characteristics. This in turn has implications for support. Parents report being labelled with attachment disorder/FII, and this arguably has potential to produce a negative effect – much as the 'refrigerator parent' term historically did for parents of autistic children.

Demand avoidance: impact on life

Demand avoidance often has a profound effect on the life of the individual and those around them. This often begins during education, with many children with demand-avoidant profiles moving from placement to placement, often following a path such as mainstream, to mainstream with support or one-to-one support, to autism specialist units, to pupil referral or behavioural units. Unfortunately, the conclusion of this path is often exclusion from formal education, with some statistics suggesting nearly 70% of children with PDA/EDA are not accessing formal education (PDA Society 2019). This continues later in life, and although research is scant, it seems to continue to pervasively impact all aspects of life including employment and relationships.

How do these differences impact the autistic birth experience?

Pregnancy, birth and the postnatal period can be stressful, emotional and painful for women in general (Hoang 2014), with estimates of around one in three women experiencing birth trauma and 4–18% reporting this has led to post-traumatic stress disorder (PTSD) resulting from the birth experience (Hill 2019a).

Women are considered vulnerable during pregnancy (Ballantyne & Rogers 2016), and autistic women may face specific challenges in childbirth due to their myriad of differences, including sensory and social differences (APA 2013).

Sensory matters (including pain)

Autistic women may have multiple sensory-processing differences, across some or all of their senses. These can include touch, taste, sound, smell, vision, spatial awareness/proprioception and balance/vestibular (Robertson & Baron-Cohen 2017). Autistic women may be hypersensitive or hyposensitive – that is, under- or over-reactive, avoidant or seeking, in terms of sensory information (Cascio *et al.* 2016). Often, they have a complicated profile, which is a mix of under- and over-sensitivity and can be complicated by other conditions that are often more common in people with autism, such as:

- **Misophonia:** A condition which triggers extreme emotional responses such as anger and/or disgust in response to an intolerance to sounds such as chewing, tapping, scratching or breathing.

- **Synaesthesia:** A condition in which an individual perceives sensory information through more than one cognitive pathway, sometimes referred to as an involuntary linking or blending of the senses (e.g. experiencing sounds such as music visually, as colours).

- **Alexithymia:** A condition which affects a person's ability to identify, process and express or describe their own feelings or the feelings of others. This can lead to confusion in differentiating between bodily sensations such as hunger or cold and emotions such as anger or sadness.

- **Hyperacusis:** A disorder of hearing where sounds can be perceived much more loudly, causing annoyance, distraction, fear, distress or even pain in the affected individual.

(Robertson & Simmons 2015; Serafini et al. 2017; Ward 2019)

In addition to these sensory differences, autistic people often have differences in interoception, something we are beginning to understand and acknowledge as the 'eighth sense' (DuBois *et al.* 2016). Interoception gathers messages from throughout our body, from multiple receptors, and our brain processes this to understand bodily sensations such as hunger, thirst, the need to urinate/defecate, temperature regulation, sexual arousal and, perhaps of key importance here, our processing and expression of pain (Hatfield *et al.* 2019).

Social interaction and communication

The diagnostic criteria for autism focus heavily on differences in social interaction, communication and imagination, and state that in order to meet the threshold for diagnosis, an individual must have pervasive issues in these areas (APA 2013; Wing, Gould & Gillberg 2011).

It is therefore unsurprising that autistic women may need differentiation in their support and could benefit from adjustments including clear communication, factual, specific and explicit information that they can relate to, processing time, visual reinforcements and, where possible, familiarisation and planning – which admittedly is restricted by the unpredictable nature of birth, but could be beneficial if implemented as far as is possible (Crane *et al.* 2018; Kennedy *et al.* 2016; Shepherd & Parry 2018).

Autistic people may struggle with social interaction, the complexities of language and non-verbal cues (Ryder 2017). Some autistic people may be non-verbal or minimally verbal, have a mismatch in expressive and receptive language or need extended processing time, all of which can have a huge impact on communication without adaptation (Ryder 2017).

Healthcare providers with limited understanding of autism may not comprehend the impact that fluctuations in functioning, affected by factors such as sensory processing, can have on the ability to interact socially and on effective communication (Donovan 2017; Nicolaidis, Kripke & Raymaker 2014).

Executive functioning, central coherence, emotional regulation

Differences in executive functioning, central coherence and emotional regulation can mean that an unfamiliar – often harsh – sensory environment coupled with an unpredictable chain of events can be hugely challenging to cope with (Kiep & Spek 2017; Lemon *et al.* 2011; Mazefsky *et al.* 2013).

Autistic women may be perceived as difficult or uncooperative when actually they are overwhelmed (Donovan 2017). Empathetic care is vital in these instances, though constraints of time/workload can make it challenging for healthcare professionals to devote additional time and energy to vulnerable patients (Hazard 2019; Hildingsson *et al.* 2018).

Autistic women face specific challenges, perhaps the most notable being the altered sensory responsivity that is said to exist in autism spectrum disorder (ASD), with multiple sensory systems affected (Robertson & Baron-Cohen 2017). Sensitivity to touch may prove the most impactful in pregnancy and childbirth, due to the jarring sensations throughout the body and the ongoing physical examinations (Riquelme, Hatem & Montoya 2016).

However, sensitivities to sight, sound and smell in a clinical environment may prove equally challenging, contributing to an overall overwhelm of the sensory systems (Hahn 2012; Nicholas *et al.* 2016).

In addition, the experience of pain may be significantly altered in autistic people (APA 2013). Sener *et al.* (2017) suggested that differences in three genes could lead to altered pain response in the autistic population, although the study was small-scale and focused entirely on children. The first fMRI study of pain responses in autistic adults – small-scale presumably due to the cost involved in this procedure, and confined to those described as high-functioning – suggested that there may be altered pain coping and evaluation in this group, although further studies are necessary to see if this generalises across the spectrum (Failla *et al.* 2017). Individuals may experience hyper- or hypo-reactivity to pain, or a combination of both, with some studies showing an abnormal response to pain in 25–40% of autistic people (Moore 2014). Researchers suggest that this altered pain sensation and reaction may account for the high levels of self-injurious behaviour in ASD (Duerden *et al.* 2013; Minshawi *et al.* 2014; Summers *et al.* 2017).

In addition to this differing perception of pain, communication of pain may also be notably different. Alexithymia is common in autism, which is an inability to identify and describe emotions in oneself and others (Costa, Steffgen & Samson 2017). Facial expressions may substantially differ, with autistic individuals suggested as presenting blunt or flat affect (Sasson & Morrison 2019). Thus, professionals may not recognise distress or pain in autistic women during labour due to this atypical presentation (Allely 2013). There is an imperative need for healthcare professionals to realise that traditional pain measurement approaches – that is, self-report and facial pain scales – may be ineffective in the autistic population. However, evidence regarding presentation of pain in autistic people is particularly conflicting, with some studies finding no difference in pain reactivity and expression (Hadjikhani *et al.* 2014; Thaler *et al.* 2017). Some studies diverge in their findings about expressivity of emotion in autistic people, possibly due to focusing on one section of the population (i.e. high-functioning) where expressivity may have been learned, or possibly simply due to the presentations of autism being as unique as the individuals themselves. In some cases, exaggerated expressions of emotion or pain may manifest, and it seems pain reactions may vary throughout life (Rattaz *et al.* 2013), so it is imperative that healthcare professionals remain open-minded to varying expressivity.

Due to the systemic differences in the sensory, nervous and immune systems in ASD, clinicians should consider that the effects of medications may also differ (Kilbaugh *et al.* 2010). Anecdotal evidence suggests that both autistic children and adults experience both hyper- and hyposensitivity to medications, though research appears very scant. A study by Li *et al.* (2017) suggested autistic people may be more sensitive to anaesthesia, although this study was limited, apparently conducted upon autistic mice. Given the complex social, emotional, mental and physiological differences between mice and humans, this finding should be viewed with some caution. Further research in this area appears warranted – ideally comparative studies on human subjects. However, if analgesia and/or sedation are shown to affect autistic people differently, this likely has a substantial effect during birth due to the intense pain mothers often experience (Van der Gucht & Lewis 2015). If a caesarean section or other surgery is needed, the effectiveness of anaesthesia is of utmost importance (Mankowitz, Gonzalez Fiol & Smiley 2016). The effects of common coexisting conditions on pain management may also have a significant impact, such as epilepsy, ADHD and other systemic conditions (Robbins & Phenicie 2011; Willner *et al.* 2014).

Studies suggest that anxiety is present in up to 84% of the autistic population (McGonigle *et al.* 2014). Other mental health conditions also appear more likely to coexist, such as depression or obsessive compulsive disorder (OCD) (Mannion & Leader 2013; Meier *et al.* 2015), as are neurodevelopmental disorders such as ADHD and dyspraxia/developmental coordination disorder (DCD) (Croen *et al.* 2015). Research suggests sleep and eating disorders may also be more prevalent, which again can impact mental, physical and emotional wellbeing (Devnani & Hegde 2015; Mandy & Tchanturia 2015). Depression and/or anxiety are often treated with selective serotonin reuptake inhibitors (SSRIs) (NICE 2009, 2011), which may be withdrawn during pregnancy due to conflicting evidence on safety of use (Du Toit *et al.* 2015), and may possibly cause an increasingly vulnerable mental and emotional state.

Research suggests autistic people have increased prevalence of other comorbidities, such as epilepsy (Thomas *et al.* 2017), autoimmune disorders, gastrointestinal problems and recurring infections (Croen *et al.* 2015; Davignon *et al.* 2018), with studies suggesting those with multimorbidity are becoming increasingly common, the number rising in England from 1.9 million in 2008 to 2.9 million in 2018 (Department of Health and Social Care 2012; King's Fund 2012). Croen *et al.* (2015) stated that diabetes and high blood pressure are twice as likely in autistic adults, with heart disease being even more common. This can lead to a complex patient profile and may be indicative of lack of or inappropriate preventative care. These conditions may also impact pain management.

Why have we overlooked the autistic birth experience?

Long has research overlooked the experience of autistic parents, including autistic women who experience sexual health, relationships, pregnancy, birth and new motherhood, as non-autistic women do (Grant 2017).

Information is so scant that upon visiting the National Autistic Society website, arguably the most prominent autism charitable organisation in the UK, you will find information pages for parents, siblings and partners of autistic people and those who have autistic parents, but at the time of writing, there is no information for autistic parents, and no information around navigating pregnancy, birth and parenthood (Fox 2022; NAS 2023).

There is very little peer-reviewed research or guidance on the experiences of autistic people who bear children (Taylor 2014). Indeed, research on sexual/reproductive issues in autistic women has long been neglected, as for women with disabilities generally (Frohmader & Ortoleva 2012).

For too long, we have thought of autism as much more prevalent in males, with a 4:1 ratio of males to females being generally referred to for some time (Fombonne 2009). Studies have varied wildly on this estimate, up to a 16:1 estimate in what some term the 'higher-functioning' autistic population. But we now know that the ratio is likely to be far closer to equal than we previously believed, with some scientists and studies suggesting a 3:1 or even 2:1 ratio.

There are several reasons for this, including theories such as extreme male brain (Baron-Cohen 2002) and the often different presentation of autism in females. Whereas males may be more likely to experience meltdown, girls are often much more internal and likely to shut down, meaning they fly under the radar and are less likely to be identified for screening, referral and assessment. This can be related back to the underlying fight, flight or freeze response in the general population that often sees fight more commonly in males, whereas flight or freeze tend to be more common among females.

We now realise that autistic females do often have the intense interests we see in males, though females often focus their intense interests on something that may be deemed 'socially acceptable' such as horses, make-up and dolls, and as such this is brushed off as typical.

Females may also focus their intense interests on reading and writing fiction – they may find comfort in characters that are undemanding and in escaping into worlds which are easier and more rewarding than reality. They often also use their intense interests to study how people think and interact, with many autistic women developing passions for fiction, psychiatry or indeed autism itself (International Society for Autism Research 2019).

There is also a male bias in our screening and diagnostic tools, and some clinicians may be inexperienced in female presentation, lacking the depth, breadth and current knowledge to interpret questions and look for more subtle signs that may point to autism in women and girls. Indeed, diagnostic interviews such as the DISCO are often better at picking up autism in females than observational tools such as the Autism Diagnostic Observation Schedule (ADOS).

Francesca Happé, director of the MRC Centre at King's College London, said of diagnosing women (Mandavilli 2015):

> Without their self-report telling you how stressful it is to maintain appearances, you wouldn't really know. They have good imitation, good intonation in their language, body language – surface behaviour isn't very useful for a diagnosis, at least for a certain set of women on the spectrum.

Females are often misdiagnosed with conditions such as anorexia and other eating disorders, anxiety disorders including social anxiety, generalised anxiety disorder, specific phobias, personality disorders and/or bipolar disorder. This is not to say these conditions cannot also be present or coexist with autism, as we will see in Chapter 3, but it is vital we investigate further when needed to avoid diagnostic overshadowing and mitigate the risk of missed or misdiagnosis.

Interestingly, the largest study to date on sex differences in executive functioning in autism found that females were rated by parents as having greater problems in executive functioning than males, also rating females as exhibiting more daily living skills difficulties (White *et al.* 2017).

Historically, women have been more likely to obtain an autism diagnosis where there is also an intellectual/learning disability (ID/LD), where they are non-verbal, and essentially where their autism is more 'visible' and observable, leading to many who may be termed 'high-functioning' to be missed or misdiagnosed (Loomes, Hull & Mandy 2017; Van Wijngaarden-Cremers *et al.* 2013; Wing 1981b).

Many women with an autism diagnosis may therefore have been

institutionalised (Goldacre, Gray & Goldacre 2015), and as a society we have a history of infantilising those with disabilities – particularly where there is a cognitive impact, viewing those with developmental conditions as 'eternal children' in many ways (Byers, Nichols & Voyer 2013; Rogers 2010). This has led to many people with these conditions not being supported to build and maintain healthy relationships and intimacy, and not receiving appropriate sexual education, though as a society we are starting to break some of the taboos around sexuality and disability, and are seeing a rise in the number of disabled women becoming pregnant and giving birth (Potvin, Brown & Cobigo 2016). Despite this, the waters remain unclear around consent, safeguarding and intervention, with concerns of forced marriage, unfair bars to marriage, and orders to allow or restrict sexual activity and to force contraception or abortion (BBC News 2019a; Buckley-Thomson 2012; Garisto Pfaff 2018; Patterson *et al.* 2018; Ryan 2017; Sawer 2018a, 2018b).

For too long we have conflated developmental delay or cognitive difference with a lack of maturity, when it could be far more beneficial to take a holistic view of a person with a 'socio scheme' and 'multiple spectrum of ages' as suggested by Delfos (2004, 2016, 2017) – see Figure 1.1. Delfos proposed that whilst in 'typical' or non-autistic development, first comes emotional development, then comes cognitive. Her belief is that this is reversed for autistic people, which could explain why it could be argued that autistic people experience and interact with the world primarily through a cognitive lens, operating more on intelligence, intellect and logic than instinct and intuition.

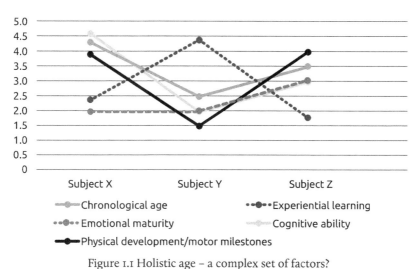

Figure 1.1 Holistic age – a complex set of factors?

This suggests that people develop differently, perhaps in a different order, with pockets of delay, acceleration and/or steady growth, making determining their 'age' much more complex than their chronological years or IQ tests would indicate. In this book, this concept has been termed 'holistic age – a complex set of factors?' with Figure 1.1 suggesting some of the potential considerations and complexities.

In recent years, we have continued to challenge our perceptions of care, of wellbeing and when it is right to intervene, realising that while complete independence is not always possible, we should still promote autonomy wherever we can (Cheak-Zamora *et al.* 2017; Hodgetts, Richards & Park 2017).

Functioning labels

It is important to remember that it is very difficult to describe an individual accurately with 'high-functioning' or 'low-functioning' labels.

The autism spectrum isn't really a line from low-functioning to high-functioning, as a lot of individuals will have high areas of ability mixed with high levels of need.

We often call extreme differences in ability and need 'spiky' profiles.

In my work on psychoeducation with autistic/neurodivergent teens, I often use the example of the *Sims* video game to explain functioning and spiky profiles. In the game, when you create a new 'sim', you have a set number of ability points you can allocate across domains such as intelligence, cleanliness, friendliness and so on. I often say that for autistic people, we tend to have high concentrations of ability points in certain domains with lower amounts in others. Essentially, I feel we are often 'calibrated differently'. A quote I live by is 'Autism lives in the extremes', which I took to saying to try to explain differences to people who struggled to understand the impact on daily life and functioning, and I feel this makes sense in many areas, like sensory seeking versus sensory avoiding, introverted versus extroverted and so on. This I believe helps explain why some autistic people have such high levels of skill mixed with such high levels of need.

Emma

Functioning labels can further reinforce this negative simplification of autistic development. They often rely on visible behaviour – 'how autistic do I look to you?' – to define someone's ability to cope, emotional and academic intelligence and need for support. This means that those autistic people who are termed 'high-functioning' often feel adrift, pressured, overlooked, with a lack of appropriate support or accommodation, while those termed 'low-functioning', which is often a perception linked to verbal or academic ability, are underestimated, even patronised, and find their autonomy reduced or removed as a consequence.

This perception of functioning is not an exclusively autistic phenomenon, rather one that often negatively impacts the wider disabled community where conditions are deemed 'invisible'.

Functioning labels are also reductive because they fail to account for the fact that functioning is variable, not static. All humans experience variations in their functioning, for example:

- **On a daily basis:** Some people are early birds who function best in the morning but find they are sleepy and less focused later in the day, while others seemingly cannot function before their coffee and work best at night. Some people may function best on a Monday, fresh from the weekend, while others take time to transition back into their workday routine.

- **Throughout the life cycle:** People often experience dips in their functioning during times of stress or change, such as a transition in education or employment, during relationship stress or divorce, when they experience a bereavement and so on.

Autistic people are more sensitive to their environment as well as to stress and change, and so our functioning may be more notably affected more often. It can do a disservice to autistic people to expect that what we can accomplish one day we can the next, and likewise to assume that because we struggle with a task one day, we will not be able to complete the said task at a different time.

Masking/camouflaging

Autistic people who mask are often referred to as 'chameleons'. They can appear to have superior superficial social skills, adapting to social situations and using mimicry to great effect in some cases.

This phenomenon is being increasingly recognised and is often referred to as 'masking' or 'camouflaging'.

Differing presentation

Common characteristics of those who mask include:

- 'blending in'
- autistic characteristics less visible
- more socially motivated
- intense interests are more 'mainstream', often focused on animals or people
- intense involvement in fiction/fantasy as escapism
- perfectionism
- overly expressive physical gestures.

> I don't like making eye contact. I do it because I have to and I know it's appropriate.
>
> *Maya, late-diagnosed autistic female*

> Some call it masking, but we call it social formatting, as in essence it's copying and pasting someone else's behaviour and trying to make it your own, but without understanding where that comes from.
>
> *Sarah Wild, Headteacher, Limpsfield Grange*

For some males, you can make a diagnosis at least provisionally in your mind within 10 minutes of them coming into your office. Whereas for some of the women, it might take half an hour or not till halfway through a diagnostic interview before they're revealing what's behind the mask.

Simon Baron-Cohen (Mandavilli 2015)

Again, the complex experience and manifestation of the phenomenon of masking is best understood from the autistic voice. Below is a poem by our author Emma on her personal experience of masking:

You tell me I 'don't look autistic',
As though I've won a prize;
When really you make it harder,
For me to let go of all the lies;
My pretence is successful,

I can almost even 'pass';
If you could see behind the curtain,
You might understand the farce;
My normalcy is faked,
A cunning rehearsed role;
It binds me and constrains me,
Stealing pieces of my soul;
I must be 'mild' you tell me,
I don't rock or flap or twirl;
My stims are much more subtle,
An elastic that I curl;
'High functioning, right?' you ask me,
As if you know what that might mean;
It means I struggle on in silence,
Hide my worries away, unseen;
I don't look autistic, you promise,
Little comfort that provides;
Because no matter how well I hide it,
I'm autistic on the inside.

Most of us alter our behaviours in some ways in different situations, or around different people, for instance, the difference between our behaviour on a first date to being married for years, or from a job interview to with a long-term colleague. Some people refer to their 'professional' mask or hat. However, this is different to the masking we are discussing here for many reasons, such as the extensiveness, pervasiveness, necessity and more. There are people from other disadvantaged groups who may mask extensively in some ways similar to that of autistic masking, such as those who are gay, trans or from ethnic minority backgrounds.

However, it is vital to remember that *not all autistic people mask.*

The extent to which someone masks, the reasons why and how they do it will all vary. The person may consciously or subconsciously mask – or a combination of both.

Are some autistic people more likely to mask than others?
In recent years, it has been increasingly acknowledged that autistic women and girls are more likely to mask – though not all women and girls mask and some boys and men do.

Some autistic people who face multiple disadvantages (intersectionality) may be more likely to mask, for instance if they are facing racial or cultural biases.

These factors can also have implications for disclosure, diagnosis, understanding and support. Autistic people may fear that diagnostic disclosure will mean losing the control that masking affords them. As we know, an autism diagnosis is based on observable behaviours demonstrated in the assessment room and is bound to this specific context (in some cases, self- and familial reporting is valid) – if a person is masking their true autistic impulses and characteristics, then it may hinder the diagnosing professional in providing a diagnosis. Many autistic women have reported that they have been required to mask for so long that their true needs and personality are difficult to unveil in public. This prompts the question of where does masking end and begin?

Where do we mask?

- School, college, university.
- Work – from interviews to meetings to everything in between.
- Social situations – as many situations that involve interacting as you can think of: parties, pub lunches, nights out, shopping, family events, leisure activities…
- Specific occasions – birthdays, weddings, Christmas, funerals.

Frankly? Everywhere. Are there other people (especially non-autistic people)? Then chances are, an autistic person uses their mask to get through that situation at some point. (Sedgewick, Hull & Ellis 2022)

The 'fizzy drink bottle effect'

This explains why someone can also present very differently in different environments – for example, at home and at school. Some describe this as the 'fizzy drink bottle effect'. It compares the difficulties throughout the day to a bottle being shaken up more and more; the contents are contained as the child does not feel safe to take off the mask. Then the 'lid comes off' and the fizzy drink 'explodes' when the child gets home. This can lead to difficulties in obtaining diagnosis and support, with parents/carers feeling disbelieved or blamed for the behaviour.

In the healthcare setting, this may manifest in a number of ways. The stoic yet labour-intensive skill of masking may mean that much of what is verbally communicated may not be absorbed and committed to medium- or long-term memory. The stress of masking may lead to a sizeable and unpleasant (to experience and observe) adrenaline 'dump' when getting home or to another safe space. The before, during and after effects of masking have psychological and physiological consequences for quite some time. For example, during antenatal observation, this may present as an increased blood pressure reading, similar to the phenomenon of 'white coat syndrome', when a person's blood pressure reading is higher in the doctor's surgery than when at home.

Why do we mask?

Every person has their own combination of factors that lead to masking, but they may include:

- survival mechanism

- stigma/lack of understanding/societal pressures

- not knowing why we are different – undiagnosed

- wanting to fit in/have friends

- not wanting to stand out/draw attention, or seem different or strange

- learned behaviour – through trauma such as bullying, negative experiences or intensive 'training'.

It's as if everybody is playing some complicated game and I am the only one who hasn't been told the rules. (Sainsbury 2000)

How do we mask?

Different types of masking

Below we list examples of types of masking (Sedgewick *et al.* 2022), but be aware that the list of types and their presentation is not exhaustive but rather a guide to the underlying mechanisms at play.

- **Instinctive:** An instinctive survival response to fear, pain, danger.

- **Ingrained:** A learned behaviour – began as a conscious choice but became embedded/conditioned (i.e. in response to certain interventions).

- **Subconscious:** A mask created in response to historical/internalised trauma.

- **Conscious/active:** Active recognition that a situation is not safe/comfortable or requires a specific way of presenting yourself.

> I think growing up and developing all these forms of masking all mashed up together can leave you confused as to who you are under the mask. I still mask both consciously and subconsciously. Sometimes I can be around someone for half an hour and go home having picked up mannerisms, speech patterns or even accent/tone of voice to some extent without realising it!
>
> *Emma*

Visible masking characteristics

- Hiding our autism – such as disguising sensory sensitivities or suppressing 'stims'.

- Becoming a 'character' – this can be quite involved and can include:

  - mimicry

  - studying other people

  - creating a persona

  - rehearsal and replays – scripts and databases and 'cross-referencing'!

- Compensating/using autistic strengths.

> I tend to compartmentalise my life quite a lot. I think part of this is I am a slightly different 'me' with each group of people, and being around them all at once would be overwhelming, which bits fit and which bits don't, even if the 'tweaks' are subtle.
>
> *Emma*

Implications of masking

Emma's words below from the autistic perspective of masking illustrate the long-term effects of this skill on the personality and wellbeing of an autistic woman:

> I remember an advert for a show called *How to Build a Girl* and the title struck a chord with me. I think I built myself over time, piece by piece, into

who I felt the world would accept. I'm working on figuring out the pieces I want to build myself with since my late diagnosis – some I'll keep and some I'll replace again bit by bit – and it feels empowering, like this time I'm in control. It's very much a work in progress, though!

Emma

Again, like diagnosis and the recognition of support needs, this is very much down to observable behaviours. The domino effect of masking can also appear as:

- exhaustion
- burnout
- low self-esteem –feeling like a failure
- physical and mental health difficulties
- risky behaviours
- victimisation
- alcohol/substance use/abuse
- loneliness.

It doesn't always work. Applying logic to human emotion and socialisation is trying to logic something that isn't logical!

It's exhausting because it's like you're doing math all day.

Kevin Pelphrey, Yale Child Study Center

If I have lots of friends but none of them see the real me, do I have any friends at all? It's like living a life of measures, and reminds me of the quote – there's nothing lonelier than feeling alone in a room full of people.

Emma

Is masking always a bad thing?

This topic may be controversial, but some autistic people say their mask can be a good thing at times in certain situations. For some of us, masking has helped us survive education, workplaces and even navigating friend-ships and relationships. The key is that someone is not compelled to mask, that they feel in control of how to use it, how often and with whom – and that they can take it off when they want to!

> After being diagnosed late, I felt a whole new sense of pressure – NOT to mask, like I was letting other autistic people down by setting a bad example of some kind. But the truth is my masks are so intertwined with who I am and have been with me for so long, I don't always know where I end and they begin even if I want or need to take them off. I'm working on letting that guard down bit by bit, but the truth is, I still need my masks to survive in a neurotypical world.
>
> *Emma*

It can take time and a lot of work to unpick masking behaviours, particularly for those diagnosed in later life. However, as research grows on the topic, we are beginning to develop tools to help with this such as the CAT-Q (described below). Using tools like the CAT-Q alongside traditional diagnostic tools can help build a fuller picture and help us measure discrepancies in external behaviours versus internal experience.

CAT-Q (Camouflaging Autistic Traits Questionnaire)

The CAT-Q measures the degree to which you use camouflaging strategies.

The more you camouflage, the more of your autistic proclivities you are likely able to suppress. As such, a high camouflaging score can also account for lower scores on other autism tests. So if you don't currently meet the diagnostic criteria but you still think you have autistic traits, this could be why.

The CAT-Q measures camouflaging in general, as well as three subcategories:

- **Compensation:** Strategies used to actively compensate for difficulties in social situations.

  Examples: Copying body language and facial expressions, learning social cues from movies and books.

- **Masking:** Strategies used to hide autistic characteristics or portray a non-autistic persona.

  Examples: Adjusting face and body to appear confident and/or relaxed, forcing eye contact.

- **Assimilation:** Strategies used to try to fit in with others in social situations.

  Examples: Putting on an act, avoiding or forcing interactions with others.

Whether you're an autistic person or someone supporting autistic people in your personal or professional life, we hope we've effectively illustrated the scope and weight of masking. You may now be wondering how you can best emancipate true autistic characteristics from the mask (if required by the autistic individual!). Below we outline some of the ways in which you can help:

Supporting someone to 'take off the mask'

- Different not less... Embrace the social model of disability and the Double Empathy Problem – these adjustments need to take place from person-centred care in the immediate context to advocating for improved understanding and patient voice in policy change.

- Recent research suggests autistic people socialise effectively with each other. The DART (Development, Autism, Research, Technology) project[3] has illustrated that autistic people share information just as effectively as neurotypical people do with one another. The ability is directly affected by understanding and accommodation, which is an incredible opportunity to help autistic parents better advocate for themselves.

- The double empathy concept. We've said it before and we'll say it again: autistic and non-autistic people are not deficient or superior versions of one another. We are wired differently but not inadequately and should be supported to embrace our identity.

- Learning each other's language.

If I went to Germany and couldn't understand people there because their language was different, I wouldn't think they were wrong or broken – just different! I would get a translation app or book, or a person to help us communicate effectively. Autism is kind of similar – it's just learning each other's language and meeting in the middle.

Emma

---

3 https://dart.ed.ac.uk

It's fair to say that masking may be a huge issue for the autistic population and a barrier to accessing the same level of healthcare as their neurotypical counterparts. While we have given a few examples of real-world masking characteristics, it's essential to understand the underlying power imbalances, stigma and other issues that may ignite the need to mask. Without this level of understanding, supporting someone who masks may fall short.

The autistic birth experience
The research landscape
There has been some limited research into the autistic birth experience, but the legacy of the medical and deficit models has meant that this is often littered with considerations about the 'risk factors' of autism. Examples of risk factors in the incidence of autism have included antidepressant use, prenatal exposure to hurricanes and grandfathers who were engineers! In the context of the neurodiversity movement, this isn't supportive and doesn't offer anything to our understanding of the autistic birth experience. Additionally, it medicalises and, in some cases, personifies the 'autistic uterus'. Rather ironically, one could argue that the neurotypical powers-that-be need to use their 'superior' central coherence ability to see the bigger picture here. As mentioned briefly above, there are emerging reports that autistic women are at higher risk of being accused of fabricated or induced illness (FII), formerly known as Munchausen's by proxy, where a mother reports or exaggerates symptoms and illnesses not confirmed by medical doctors. Some report that this is due to the complex nature of co-occurring and autism presentations; others have argued the higher proportion of autistic women with health anxiety may be a factor. Regardless of the cause, we need to understand the preconceptions of autistic mothers before we interpret any research on the topic.

Furthermore, there is a long history of infantilising disabled sexuality and womanhood. Autism awareness may increase, but we are still not at the point where we know enough due to the legacy of deficit models, stigma and lack of holistic quality-of-life consideration in the appreciation of alternative measurements and priorities of the autistic community.

Historically, autistic people, as part of the disabled community, have experienced stigma around sexual desire and identity (Salà *et al.* 2019). This stigma may still today affect the autistic experience in pubertal transitioning to adulthood, with the potential to be compounded by core aspects of autism such as social communication and interaction deficits (Beggiato *et al.* 2017); which may impact how they initiate or perceive these relationships and subsequent boundaries. The autistic community has also reported that, for some, sexual intimacy or physical contact of any kind can become overwhelming for sensory limits (Milner *et al.* 2019). While the current landscape has embraced neurodiversity and is adapting to the female presentation of autism, there is an evidenced lack of support available throughout an autistic woman's lifespan (Milner *et al.* 2019).

Autistic women are far more likely to have experienced childhood trauma, sexual assault and abuse, domestic violence and bullying, particularly in the formative teen years (Roberts *et al.* 2015), and this can impact their ability to accessing sufficient gynaecological and obstetrical care.

There is a need for tailored education beginning with family planning/ sexual health education for autistic people starting during the teen years. Often, an autistic person may need more specific information about how their body works, the impact of puberty, understanding intimacy and consent, which may not be readily available across the board. Often the burden of providing this kind of specific, specialised, tailored information falls to the parents/carers, and some may struggle with the intensity and ethics of how and when to have these conversations. Particularly where there are developmental differences, it can be difficult to reconcile a young person who in certain ways may seem 'younger' than their peers with a developing potentially sexual being. As a subject that has long been overlooked, there is a lack of information about how autism affects intimacy generally. For example, sensory sensitivities may mean that intimacy requires specific accommodations or adjustments to make it comfortable and enjoyable for both the autistic person and their sexual partner. Put simply, sex is a 'messy business', which can prove challenging for autistic people, although they may not realise why until much later in life, if at all. In relation to individual support, many other life transition events are better documented, including published materials and courses to help the support network on matters such as puberty, changing school and starting employment. However, on the topic of pregnancy and birth, such robust support and training is not widely available to the layperson.

Research has found that while, overall, autistic girls reported more confidence in their ability to maintain new hygiene routines and 'cope' with bodily changes, parents' reports did not adhere to this and reported lower confidence in these matters (Cummins, Pellicano & Crane 2020). However, no research was found that could gauge which was more accurate, giving an unclear picture of puberty transition 'success'.

Mirroring much of the medical model discourse around autism, autism research literature often focuses on 'risk factors' for the incidence of autism rather than person-centred best practice. The idea of 'preventing' autism isn't in line with the growing neurodiversity movement and, anecdotally, many female autistic advocates reject the notion. It is fair to say that for the autistic birth experience, applying both the medical and social models of disability would be most fitting to holistically engage autistic individuals during the birth experience.

The medicalisation of autistic birth, in terms of risks and complications, can be argued to be necessary due to the complex nature of autism. Furthermore, there are a number of co-occurring conditions more prevalent in the autistic population (e.g. communication issues, learning difficulties, epilepsy, ADHD and digestive problems). There is also emerging evidence that the female autistic population has additional associated health issues such as Ehlers–Danlos syndrome, chronic fatigue syndrome (CFS)/myalgic encephalomyelitis (ME), fibromyalgia and other chronic pain conditions. This is essential to consider when faced with the limited research on the autistic birth experience. Evidence from Autistica (2016) suggests that being autistic alone is a factor for poor mental health as autistic people are nine times more likely to die by suicide than non-autistic people due to the cumulative effects of bullying, exclusion, unemployment and inaccessible mental healthcare. Pregnancy itself increases the risk of depression for up to 20% of all women, which increases again if a pre-existing mental health condition is apparent (Shakespere 2015). Given that suicide is, at the time of writing, the leading cause of maternal death (Knight *et al.* 2022), it follows that autistic women are at a higher risk of developing depression and therefore may need support early in the perinatal period. This is essential for the health and wellbeing of the parents and also the unborn baby in terms of attachment and bonding. Whether from a medical or social model perspective, needs are unlikely to be identified if relevant medical professionals lack the fundamental knowledge and awareness of such conditions.

As previously discussed, autistic people process and perform gender differently to their non-autistic peers. Many report issues with 'performing' as a female, which may be related to masking habits from copying role models or a lifelong sense of gender dysphoria. Failing to take this into account may cause trauma if the patient has a difference in connecting to their female body and the physical act of giving birth. Additionally, autistic women are far more likely to have experienced childhood trauma, sexual assault and abuse, domestic violence and bullying in the formative teen years. Acknowledging these issues could facilitate improved consent and safety for the autistic individual.

This may have genuine repercussions for the birth process when considered as a potential invasion of consent, human rights and equality law. Furthermore, pain processing and communication differences render this subject a matter of urgency. Research suggests that autistic individuals process pain differently, their skin having hypersensitivity whether to touch from another person or to fabric (Griffin OT 2018). The neurological response to pain stimulus also serves to intensify the already evidenced hypoactivity in the motor and limbic cortices, resulting in 'shutdown' or the inability to communicate (both verbally and physically).

As previously mentioned, many autistic women report a lack of support for life events such as teen transition, romantic relationships, employment and retirement. However, the event of birth and becoming a parent has far-reaching consequences throughout one's natural life. The physical, emotional and mental wellbeing of the autistic mother is central, but so too are the needs of the wider family network.

Current research

Interest seems to be growing on the topic of 'autistic birth', with its inclusion on the agenda at the NAS Women and Girls Conference 2019 in Edinburgh, and a PhD project by Autistica (King 2019). Cambridge University's Autism Research Centre has been doing some research in this area for the past few years, but unfortunately it seems to have drifted into focusing on early identification of autism in the uterus, which has concerning ethical implications for prevention, cure and termination (Cox 2014).

It is increasingly accepted that autistic women have been overlooked in diagnosis, research and support (Bargiela, Steward & Mandy 2016). Our screening and diagnostic tools and, indeed, our understanding of autism itself have evolved from the observation of males (Krahn & Fenton 2012), thus missing not only autistic women but also many who have other disabilities/co-occurring conditions, those do not fit the binaries of gender or sexuality and those from other ethnicities, cultures and socioeconomic backgrounds (Donohue *et al.* 2017; Durkin et al. 2017; Harrison *et al.* 2017; NAS 2014; Newschaffer 2017; Yingling, Hock & Bell 2018).

It is ironic in some ways that the intersectionality of autism and these other marginalised groups has led to confusion and dismissal, as we are now beginning to understand that autistic people are more likely to belong to the LGBTQIA+ community, experience gender variances (George & Stokes

2017; Jacobs *et al.* 2014; Janssen, Huang & Duncan 2016; Stagg & Vincent 2019; Strang *et al.* 2014) and have co-occurring conditions/disabilities than the general population (Croen *et al.* 2015; Findon *et al.* 2016).

Women have often not only been 'missed' but misdiagnosed, often with conditions such as eating disorders, anxiety, depression, bipolar or personality disorders (Kirkovski, Enticott & Fitzgerald 2013; Mandy & Tchanturia 2015). That is not to say these conditions cannot coexist with autism, and, indeed, emerging research suggests they often do (Mandy & Tchanturia 2015; Hambrook *et al.* 2008; Rosen *et al.* 2018), but they are sometimes erroneously diagnosed or cause diagnostic overshadowing, leading to an autism diagnosis being exceedingly difficult to come by for some women (Lai, Baron-Cohen & Buxbaum 2015). Cambridge Autism Research Centre's (ARC) paper reported feedback from an advisory panel of 355 autistic mothers (91 of whom were parents of autistic children without a diagnosis themselves) (Pohl *et al.* 2020). Autistic mothers were more likely to report greater difficulties with accessing social events with/for their child and feelings of isolation and depression. There were participant concerns about stigma, such as feeling judged for parenting ability and not being understood by medical professionals (Hampton *et al.* 2022). The research recommended better tailored support during pregnancy and postnatally. This is pertinent for autistic mothers and mothers of children with autism, who are more likely to have contact with social services and be accused of FII (Davis, Murtagh & Glaser 2019). However, as so much of autism and pregnancy research is risk-based or deficit-lensed, researchers must explicitly refute this is an aim of their work if they are to be considered neuro-affirming (Pohl *et al.* 2020):

> autistic women provide the uterine environment for their baby, and this may contain a number of important uterine environmental factors that interact with an increased genetic likelihood of developing autism. These include the metabolic pathways associated with gestational diabetes, including insulin and testosterone exposure to the fetus.

It may be argued that the concept of a pathologised 'autistic uterus' and connotations of the extreme male brain theory (Baron-Cohen 2002; Baron-Cohen, Leslie & Frith 1985; Hanley *et al.* 2015) potentially having long-term implications for wellbeing is not coherent with the socially driven results of the survey. Furthermore, while results are largely social model-based and somewhat reflect anecdotal calls for more social support from autistic parents, the mention of risk/incidence factors is questionable. The survey featured several rating scale questions focused on the anger levels of autistic mothers during and after pregnancy.

The realities of the social stigma and isolation reported in the survey are arguably a valid causal link to maternal feelings of anger. Additionally, from a medical perspective, the involvement of cortisol and adrenaline produced in stressful events may provide further scope for research on stress levels in autistic women. This would enable researchers to fully investigate the potential role played by endocrine activity, whether causal or symptomatic. Potvin *et al.* (2016) provide a relevant framework for the perception of support available for women with intellectual and developmental disabilities. Three main factors were identified, with effects on perception of care from the autistic population:

> (1) support is accessible, (2) support is provided by individuals expressing positive attitudes towards the pregnancy, and (3) autonomy is valued. (Potvin *et al.* 2016)

Although evidence thus far has suggested pregnancy-specific care for autistic individuals is somewhat lacking, some good practice has been implemented (although at this stage there is no peer review of these initiatives). For example, a Maternity and Infant Care result found Henry's (2017) resources created for pregnant autistic women in Suffolk, published at the time by Leeds Health Board. Henry (2017) offers a 'Pregnancy Passport' with the aim of communicating the pregnant woman's needs, covering common issues such as consent over touch during observations, sequencing of events and pain communication. Two earlier versions of the passport encompassed a text version and another, using visual prompts, created by Leeds and York Partnership service called 'easy on the i' (Leeds and York Partnership NHS Foundation Trust 2023). The idea was for women to use the passport during pregnancy, with support if required, to convey their care preferences. The acknowledgment of the higher likelihood of mothers who have been subjected to sexual abuse or trauma is served with questions such as 'I am happy to have males involved in my care'; sensory/consent issues include 'I would like to wear my own clothes in labour' (Henry 2017). Links to photographs of the hospital are provided, which may well lessen the fear of an unknown environment, reported as a barrier to maternity admissions of autistic patients (Symon 2017). This could be improved by providing photographs of key staff members likely to be involved in care, as autistic people often have difficulty reading or remembering faces (Stantić *et al.* 2021).

During 2019, the passports were developed further with support from the Florence Nightingale Foundation and the East Suffolk and North Essex Foundation Trust (ESNEFT 2021). The passport was developed into three separate support plans to encompass the antenatal, intrapartum and post-natal period (Henry 2022, 2023). As the project was funded by a hospital trust, one of the specifications was for the plans to be simplified to be more inclusive for people with a learning disability. This meant that the text-only version was replaced with visual plans, which autistic people may or may not be offended by, given the simplicity of the plans and the connotations this may present for them. The plans were implemented in March 2020 which, sadly, coincided with the Covid-19 outbreak and so the plans were introduced at a time when mandatory staff training had been suspended. This meant that the plans were only implemented within a specialist team who supported autistic women with co-occurring difficulties such as poor mental health, learning disabilities and social issues antenatally and postna-tally, but not during their hospital admission; therefore, staff working in the hospital were not aware of the plans' contents or how to make adjustments to care. The plans have been taken up by the East Suffolk and North Essex integratory health board, who hope to roll the plans out alongside training for staff in the East of England; however, the plans can be downloaded and used elsewhere (Henry 2022). Although the plans promote autonomy for birthing people to be forthright about their support needs, there is no legal obligation for hospitals to use them yet.

Previous studies have suggested that reported examples of autistic autonomy have been misinterpreted by staff as aggressive, and direct lan-guage as 'too black-and-white'. Arguably, a woman armed with this passport may risk being negatively perceived by some staff. Ideally, there is a need for documents and protocols to legally bind staff to gauge and adapt their own skills when caring for autistic women. Furthermore, during times of austerity, poor staffing levels and wait times need to be considered when advising new practices.

In some cases, women may not see the same midwife regularly, making allocating a specialist difficult. Overall, these documents show promise and could be adopted in most health boards due to the low cost of production. However, as it stands, legally in Wales the Autism Plan covers non-devolved matters, suggesting a NICE pathway may address the issues faced by autistic women becoming mothers by providing a unified, accountable framework for all devolved nations in the United Kingdom. Any guideline would need to consider the social model of disability and explore the disabling impact that clinical medicalised environments can have for some autistic people. This could be achieved by co-producing the guideline with autistic people.

What are the potential results of this lack of awareness, understanding and support?

It is often useful to give consideration to Oliver's (1997) social model of disability (see Figure 1.2), framed helpfully by Beardon's (2018) 'Autism + Environment = Outcome'. This idea suggests we can reduce the level of disability, distress and deterioration someone experiences based on appropriate support; conversely, failure to provide appropriate support and outcomes can cause significant negative impact and an increase in the level of disability someone experiences (Woods 2017).

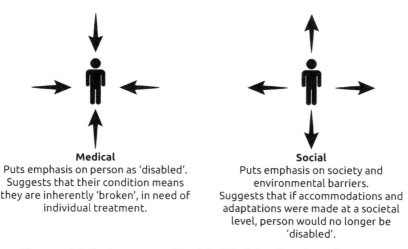

Medical
Puts emphasis on person as 'disabled'. Suggests that their condition means they are inherently 'broken', in need of individual treatment.

Social
Puts emphasis on society and environmental barriers. Suggests that if accommodations and adaptations were made at a societal level, person would no longer be 'disabled'.

Figure 1.2 Medical versus social model of disability (based on Oliver 1997)

> I read an analogy that really relates to Autism + Environment = Outcome which resonated strongly with me. Written by an autistic blogger, it sug-gested that we compare autistic and neurotypical people to saltwater and freshwater fish. If you take a saltwater fish and place it in a freshwater fish tank, it may struggle to swim and breathe and may even die. But it is not the fish that is faulty; it is the environment that is inhospitable. If we reversed the scenario and placed a freshwater fish in a saltwater fish tank, the same outcome is likely to occur. So since I read that blog, I tend to think of autistic people as 'minority fish in a neurotypical world'.
>
> *Emma*

There are many significant potential outcomes of a lack of appropriate support, including a higher likelihood of intervention, complications and trauma (Rönnerhag *et al.* 2018). There is also the potential for post-traumatic stress disorder post childbirth (PTSD-PC) for both the woman and her partner/loved ones, which can have a negative impact on bonding with the infant and thus, potentially, child development, as well as negatively impacting relationships (Patterson *et al.* 2018).

For some women, who may very much want children, their fear of pregnancy and childbirth – tokophobia – becomes so overwhelming that without appropriate support they feel unable to pursue their dreams of motherhood or further children (Brouwer *et al.* 2018; Patterson *et al.* 2018; Striebich, Mattern & Ayerle 2018; Teixeira & Machado 2016). Autistic women have stated that they feel unable to cope with the sensory challenges, the idea of a 'parasite' inside them and the stress of such a medicalised experience (Kim 2014a, 2014b; Phillips 2019). However, the right to family life is an essential human right (European Convention on Human Rights 1953; Human Rights Act 1998) and, medically and morally, we should support women to reduce anxiety, increase information and allow them to make informed, balanced choices based on their wishes and capabilities rather than fear or lack of support (Birthrights 2013; WHO 2018).

Other specific phobias which may have links to sensory sensitivities and/or anxiety, such as emetophobia, could also cause additional difficulties during pregnancy. Emetophobia is an intense fear of vomiting which could make morning sickness, or even the prospect of morning sickness, difficult or even impossible to contemplate, even without complicating conditions such as hyperemesis gravidarum, which causes excessive nausea and vomiting during pregnancy, at play.

What can we do to improve the experience and outcomes of autistic women and their loved ones?

It is clear from the research that enhanced knowledge and understanding often equals enhanced empathy and thus better quality of care (Haque 2019; Howick & Rees 2017; Moloney & Gair 2015). Professionals often do want to help but do not know best how to do this or are afraid of 'getting it wrong' (Nicolaidis *et al.* 2015; Preißmann 2017; Zerbo *et al.* 2015). There is much to be done in improving the experiences of pregnancy, birth and parenting for autistic people and their loved ones, and perhaps most key is provision of training that means healthcare workers have at minimum a baseline understanding of the neurotype, characteristics, behaviours and, more importantly, potential drivers of behaviours, communication and how they can make reasonable adjustments to better accommodate these differences.

Redshaw *et al.* (2013) found that while disabled women accessed their pregnancy 'booking' appointment at comparable timeframes to their non-disabled peers, across antenatal services overall, they were more likely to engage with significantly more contact (e.g. 34% of autistic women having ten or more checks, compared with 21% in the non-disabled population). However, Mitra *et al.* (2015) found that UK women with intellectual delay or disability were 'less likely to receive prenatal care' during this time. Additionally, fewer disabled women accessed antenatal classes (53%) than their peers (62%) (Redshaw *et al.* 2013). This suggests that initial booking/monitoring appointments may be more accessible, with those based on socialising harder to access. This may be due to autistic characteristics such as problems navigating new journeys alone, meeting new people or engaging in social chat (Lahiri *et al.* 2013; Schmit *et al.* 2000).

This was echoed by Beebe and Gossler (2013), who found that autistic women who did initiate and maintain friendships in pregnancy reported that those relationships with other mothers were restricted too. Furthermore, there is a concerning reflection of midwifery attitudes: 'Personally, I am comfortable with a woman with autism being pregnant; however, I was aware that not everybody held the same viewpoint as me' and 'with some care providers reporting feelings of shock, disbelief or revulsion' (Taylor 2014).

However, Taylor (2014) does acknowledge how such reactions may negatively affect the care such professionals provide to autistic women (McKay-Moffat 2007 cited in Taylor 2014). Furthermore, Mitra *et al.* (2015) reported that Irish pregnant women with intellectual or developmental disabilities welcomed pregnancy, but their healthcare providers viewed them as 'high risk liabilities'.

Xie and Gemmill (2018) reported a discord between patient and physician reporting of autonomous and successful parenting abilities, with social services becoming involved in 14 of 15 cases where the woman had intellectual or developmental disabilities. While pregnancy and birth are a time of great transition for any woman, as previously discussed, there are several characteristics of autism or co-occurring conditions that may impact the ability to access quality care and autonomy. One of the very early signs of pregnancy, morning sickness, may be complicated by pre-existing interoceptive and proprioceptive difficulties that make recognising morning sickness or accommodating morning sickness remedies more difficult (Rogers *et al.* 2017). For example, comorbidities such as eating disorders, avoidant/restrictive food intake disorder (ARFID) and limited diets are more likely to impact diet pre-pregnancy (Lucarelli *et al.* 2017). Furthermore, Rogers *et al.* (2017) noted that morning sickness and bodily changes during pregnancy may add to an already existing state of sensory overload, further compounded by the challenges of communicating this issue to health professionals. Conducting a review of blogs by autistic mothers about pregnancy and parenting, they quoted a mother concerned with sensory stress: 'I seemed able to cope...until people started to touch me.'

This brings into focus the issues mentioned above in terms of autonomy, consent and sensory overwhelm. During the physical examinations required in pregnancy, many of the reports mentioned recommended best practice for this.

Many academics believe such inequalities are rooted in long-standing issues that began with the very conceptualisation of autistic experiences. Many, including Kanner, Asperger, Frith and Baron-Cohen, produced research with what is now considered to be predominantly a male-biased lens. Many of the case studies were young, white male autistic people, which, it is argued, has led to gender and racial biases in autism research and, consequently, public narratives.

One of the best-known activists to champion the female presentation of autism is Dr Temple Grandin, an autistic American professor of animal behaviour studies. In the UK, autistic advocates such as Tania Marshall, Lana Grant, Sara Hendrickx and Dr Wenn Lawson have further contributed to the emerging profile of varied gender presentation in the autistic population.

A recent report by George and Stokes (2017) suggested that autistic women are 30 times more likely to be non-heterosexual in comparison with their typically developing peers. Furthermore, non-typical gender presentation is more prevalent in the autistic community, which may impact upon access to appropriate care provision.

While the current landscape has embraced neurodiversity and is adapting to the female presentation of autism, there is an evidenced lack of support available throughout an autistic woman's lifespan. Giving birth is undoubtedly one of the biggest transitions a woman may experience. It is well known that autistic people struggle with transition periods, and it is of great concern that this transition to becoming a parent remains inadequately managed (Heyworth *et al.* 2023; Hwang & Heslop 2023; Marriott *et al.* 2022).

A brief history of childbirth practice, culture and autonomy

Similar to autism research, midwifery practice has long been dominated by the presence of a dichotomy between the medical and social models of health alongside a male-lensed bias. This section will concurrently explore how maternity care and perspectives of disability have been shaped throughout history.

Women and birthing people have long been cared for throughout the perinatal period by a midwife. As a practice, midwifery first appears in the ancient Egyptian Ebers Papyrus around 1550 BC. The name itself derives from the Anglo-Saxon era meaning 'with woman' (Kitzinger 1991) and is a term which signals a professional identity, women-centred practice and a partnership with women (Bradfield *et al.* 2019).

Holding a low status due to being 'women's work', midwives historically struggled to rise in a male-dominated world by being excluded from medical schools in the third century and branded as witches by the medieval churches during the 14th, 15th and 16th centuries (Coleman 1985). Before the 17th century, all areas of medicine except midwifery were male dominated, until several men began to take an interest in the care of pregnant women. From the 17th century onwards, male midwives and surgeons argued that their self-proclaimed inherent superiority in technical skills enabled them to provide women with a safer service and so, from this point, the male-dominated approach to childbirth care began. Female midwives were required to conform and, in many cases, despite their more advanced expertise, became doctors' assistants; doctors carried 'greater prestige by virtue of their profession and gender' (Kitzinger 1991).

The same time period saw shifts in the understanding of disability as English society began to place less importance on the religiously dominated perspective from the Tudor period. Working-class disabled people often lived in the communities, where they worked, married and supported themselves. The cause of disability had begun to move from being God-given or rooted in an astrological cause, to being misfortunate, and worthy of charity if the disabled person was destitute. Madness moved from being rooted in possession of the soul by paranormal forces to a loss of reason. The latter could be treated; for example, reason could be restored with treatment (Jarrett 2012). Therefore, the 18th century saw the rise of hospitals in general and the rise of asylum institutions for people deemed to be disabled or 'unfit' at the time. Definitions included incurably sick, disabled aged veterans of war, deaf and dumb, epileptics and lunatics. These people were likely to be taken from their communities and housed in mostly terrible and cruel living conditions (Historic England 2022; Lee 2007).

It could be retrospectively argued that some of those admitted to asylums had a learning disability or were possibly autistic. Despite prevailing opinion, autism is not a product of modern civilisation or a new phenomenon. Historically, autism has potentially been hidden under labels such as brain damage, schizophrenia and even eccentricity, where the bearers of such labels were relegated to the margins of society (Silberman 2015). Ironically, it is noted that many such asylums housed a higher proportion of women than men despite the opposite being reflected in the general population's sex ratio. This is demonstrated in the 1871 census which shows a ratio of male-to-female asylum patients of 1000:1242 when the general population had a ratio of 1056:1000 (Appignanesi 2008). This possibly coincided with the Lunatics Act of 1845 which offered free provision for the poor; some historians have argued that it could be related to the medicalisation of maternity care.

During the 18th and 19th centuries, the rising middle classes began to prefer obstetric care over the care of a traditional midwife. This has been attributed to the fact that this choice aligned with a perceived higher social status, a factor that arguably had more bearing on quality-of-life measures than today's measures of literacy, healthcare access and housing. Birth in hospitals with babies delivered by doctors did not make childbirth any safer; in fact, Kitzinger (1991) argues that almost as many women died in 1903 (4 per 1000) as they had 50 years earlier (6 per 1000 in 1847). Birth at this time was safer at home with a Victorian midwife than in the 'lying-in hospitals' providing inpatient care. This was because 40% of maternal deaths were caused by puerperal fever, an infection now attributed to doctors moving between patients and the mortuary and delivering babies without washing their hands (Carter & Duriez 1986). Showalter (1987) suggests that at this time, around 7–10% of female asylum admissions were of women suffering from puerperal fever; therefore, women who did survive childbirth in the hospital had a good chance of being admitted to an asylum through no fault of their own. Interestingly, women were also admitted to asylums during this time for 'mania in pregnancy, fright in childbirth, puerperal mania/

insanity, insanity of lactation, and mania caused by iron deficiency anaemia and malnourishment' (Campbell 2020; Tobia 2017).

On closer inspection of the 'conditions' listed, all apart from iron-deficiency anaemia would now be referred to as postnatal depression or postpartum psychosis. Today, maternity provision offers screening for such things, not to prevent 'mania' but to support physical and mental health. Women are offered many blood tests during pregnancy, one of which tests haemoglobin levels, where a low level could indicate iron-deficiency anaemia. Haemoglobin levels may be tested again following birth, depending on the amount of blood lost or the woman's physical symptoms at the time. Iron-deficiency anaemia can be treated in a variety of ways depending upon the severity of the deficiency. Some women will be advised to eat iron-rich foods; others may be offered iron tablets, an iron transfusion or possibly a blood transfusion, especially if there are symptoms such as tachycardia, breathlessness or feeling weak, fatigued or dizzy. Anaemia would certainly not be treated by a trip to an asylum as it was for women historically. Similarly, midwives enquire about women's mental health at every contact, and most health trusts have a designated perinatal mental health service for women experiencing deterioration in mood during pregnancy or depression during the postnatal period. Some women do require hospitalisation for poor mental health, especially those who experience postnatal psychosis; however, there is a greater emphasis of early detection and support than there was in the past. The system is not perfect; there is a lot more work to be done.

It is also interesting to note how the Victorian feminine ideal of a passive, compassionate wife and mother at the centre of the family was used as a means to admit women to the asylum for undesirable behaviours such as minor eccentricity or excitability, talking too much, a disinterest in children or rejection of the family and the mothering role. Given that autistic women can appear to behave outside of the societal norm, it may be that autistic women were admitted to asylums if they did indeed survive childbirth.

At the close of the 19th century, mortality rates of mothers and babies remained unchanged. Despite several reports into the uncleanliness of hospitals, mortality became redefined as a social problem, which led to a movement for community clinical and antenatal care (Oakley 1984). This turnaround demonstrates how 19th-century doctors and male midwives believed mortality rates could be lowered simply by removing birth from women's homes. However, such moves arguably added to mortality rates through unhygienic practices. Then, when no change to mortality was noted, the 'problem' was placed back into society almost as if they washed their hands of the issue, but not quite.

Around the same time, changes were afoot for lay midwives, which began to be influenced by social class. The Matron's Aid Society was formed in 1881 (almost immediately changing its name to the Midwives Institute) and managed by several well-educated women volunteers. The society later became the Royal College of Midwives (RCM) which still exists today. The aim of the society was to recruit well-educated young women who would gain professional midwifery status and replace the 'ignorant, untrained' working-class labour force 'who were a danger to mothers and babies' (Robinson & Thompson 1995). The membership rules were so strict, however, that only 25 midwives were registered in 1895. In 1902, the first Midwives Act passed with the intent of eradicating the untrained midwives practising through the introduction of a register; however, the RCM had to lower the criteria somewhat in order to reach 1000 registrants by 1908 (Robinson & Thompson 1995). Despite the lowered criteria, the cost of midwifery training was too expensive for most working-class women, and examinations were written in medical Latin, so it was almost impossible for a woman from any social class to become a midwife (Leap & Hunter 2013).

The early 20th century saw political pressure on the government to set up schemes for maternity and child welfare (Campbell & Macfarlane 1994). By 1890, 98.7 % of births were in the home, 1% took place in workhouse infirmaries (for those who were too poor or ill to support themselves), and 0.3% took place in voluntary hospitals or 'lying-in' maternity hospitals (Campbell & Macfarlane 1994). By 1915, local authorities and voluntary societies were given grants to provide home visiting for expectant mothers, maternity centres for antenatal and infant care clinics and the provision of in patient beds within maternity homes. The emphasis of maternity homes was not on safety but reflected the fact that many people lived in homes unsuitable for birth (Campbell & Macfarlane 1994). Although the expectation for the maternity homes was high, mortality rates did not reduce. By the early 1920s, 50 new maternity homes with more than 500 beds had been provided by local authorities and voluntary agencies, with schemes in progress to provide a further 20 homes with 250 beds. However, many authorities extended their infirmaries to offer maternity services to paying patients (Campbell & Macfarlane 1994), where middle-class women assumed that higher fees ensured better care standards (Leap & Hunter 2013).

During the 1920s and 1930s, campaigns for institutional care were organised by different sources, including the Women's Co-Operative Guild who emphasised the unfit conditions of most working-class women's homes and the need for ten days' rest following birth. Obstetricians stressed the clinical need for women to give birth in hospital because it was considered safer, while middle-class women campaigned for anaesthesia. However, in 1936, the British Medical Association deemed childbirth to be 'normal' not 'clinical' and stated that 'birth can more safely be conducted at home than in hospital' (Campbell & Macfarlane 1994). By 1937, the number of women having babies in institutions had risen from 15% in 1927 to 34.8%, which led the Royal College of Obstetricians and Gynaecologists (RCOG) to recommend that maternity accommodation should be provided to allow 70% of births to occur in hospital; ten years later, they called for all births to take place in a hospital.

With the implementation of the National Health Service (NHS) in 1948, hospital births became more popular and, in some parts of the country, demand outstripped supply. The target of 70% of births taking place in institutions was achieved in 1964; however, this rise coincided with a fall in the number of births taking place overall (Campbell & MacFarlane 1994). By 1992, 96.5% of all births occurred in an NHS obstetric unit while only 1.3% of babies were born at home, so the original aims of the RCOG were almost met by 1992. Despite birth moving from home to hospital, maternal mortality did not decrease dramatically. The rate in 1910–1912 was 3.95 per 1000 and was still 3.29 per 1000 in 1940–1942. A decrease to 0.88 per 1000 was apparent by 1950–1952 (Wisniewski 2000), which can probably be attributed to the implementation of NHS standardisation of care where women received antenatal and postnatal care and therefore may have been healthier.

Bringing the midwifery story forward to today, it would be unfair to compare maternal mortality rates against rates 75–100 years ago because women's lives are very different today. Health is much more than life-or-death, and midwifery care focuses on health promotion through the salutogenesis approach, which simply means examining the origins (genesis) of health. Compared to the past, there is greater awareness today of determinants of physical and mental health (WHO 2017). These determinants include income, gender, social networks, employment, culture, genetics, housing, educational attainment and a developing awareness of how healthcare is inequitable for neurodiverse and autistic people (Henry 2022). Evidence demonstrates that autistic people have significantly poorer physical and mental health plus a lowered life expectancy (Bishop-Fitzpatrick & Kind 2017). This is not because they are autistic, but rather that this factor directly correlates with inaccessible healthcare and lack of support (Henry 2023; Mason *et al.* 2019). Society grows and changes culturally; nevertheless, maternity services still focus on preventing maternal and infant mortality and use this as a factor to inform future care recommendations (HSIB 2022; MBRRACE-UK 2021; NHS England 2019b).

Currently, almost all women in England and Wales give birth in a hospital (97.9% in 2019) (Brigante 2022), although this does not necessarily mean that the remaining 2.1% give birth at home, as this figure also includes babies born in car parks, in ambulances or on holiday, and those who freebirth, which means giving birth without the presence of a midwife (Hall 2021). Pregnancy and birth are categorised in terms of risk and treated as medical events, and only hindsight can determine whether this was necessary or not. Two truths simultaneously exist in the realm of pregnancy and birth: the first is that pregnancy and birth are not medical events, and the second is that some pregnancies and births can be medical events (Spain 2022). It could be argued that society is losing sight of the first truth, with birth being heavily influenced by medical processes and interventions to prevent mortality, such as ultrasounds and foetal monitoring, and measured by variables such as age, weight, medical conditions and ethnicity (Clesse *et al.* 2018). Indeed, the race to prevent stillbirth is no longer a debate about the place of birth but rather the method and timing of birth, which is demonstrated through the rising and alarming rates of intervention. Between 2021 and 2022, 578,562 babies were born in the UK. Of this number only 47% went into labour spontaneously; 33% of women had their labours induced and 20% underwent a caesarean section. Of the women who laboured, only 53% experienced a vaginal birth, with 12% experiencing an instrumental birth and 35 % undergoing a caesarean section (NHS 2022).

This modern approach is described by Wickham (2021) as 'the technocratic paradigm', whereby childbirth is pathologically risk-laden and needs monitoring and interventions from those who know best. It can be argued that any issue deemed a medical condition will attract the same narrative – indeed, autism itself is surrounded by similar dehumanising, deficit-based language. The point is knowing when to stop and look at how far down the wrong road one is travelling. The focus has been on mortality for so long that morbidity is increasing in response. Although not all maternity professionals subscribe to this way of thinking, and, indeed, some women do genuinely need medical support, intervention is embedded as a norm within maternity care and is certainly reflected in statistics surrounding onset of labour and method of birth (NHS 2022).

From the moment a woman finds herself pregnant, her pregnancy is calculated, measured and managed against guidelines and algorithms that offer little evidence for their use. One example of this is the 'due date', which is not a 'best before' date or a 'give birth by' date; it is an approximate date on which only 5% of babies are born, yet it is a date that is used to dictate the entire pregnancy (Wickham 2021). Due dates are often assigned to women by machines (scans) or professionals; women's own knowledge is rarely considered, despite them often knowing the date of conception or the length of their menstrual cycle. Working in this way conveys the ideal that science knows far more than the woman, her own body and that of her baby. This, according to Wickham (2021), is the epitome of the enlightenment ideal whereby the 'men who do science can control nature'.

The origin of the due date is a topic of debate. The earliest written record of pregnancy length originates around 2400 years ago with Aristotle and the suggestion that pregnancy is ten lunar months. This was interpreted as being 280 days based on the significance of the numbers 7 and 40 (Elverdam & Wielandt 1994) and never based on observation or research (Wickham 2021). In 1709, Dutch doctor Hermann Boerhaave created the algorithm still in use today of adding 7 days and 9 months to the last menstrual period (LMP). This algorithm was reported by Naegele in 1830 and is often referred to as 'Naegele's rule'. Neither Boerhaave nor Naegele documented whether the estimated pregnancy period should begin from the end of the menstrual period or from the start, but obstetric textbook authors decided it should be the latter. This means that the non-evidence-based pregnancy length estimate may be shorter than originally intended, which has indeed been proven through research (Wickham 2021). It is suggested that measuring gestational length at the time was a means of proving paternity rather than supporting maternal and foetal wellbeing. Doctors were called upon to prove whether enough time had elapsed between sex and birth (Saunders & Paterson 1991). Women were not listened to even then, as doctors could override their knowledge with their own and be bribed by an alleged father to do so (Wickham 2021).

The due date calculated from the LMP is used initially to determine when a woman should be scanned. At this scan, the due date is often changed because the scanning machine is programmed with the theory that the size of the foetus equals the length of pregnancy (Wickham 2021). This theory is also inaccurate for at least one in three women, because foetal growth varies as a range and is not fixed. This was proven by Källén *et al.* (2013), who measured babies conceived by IVF on a guaranteed date and found variation in foetal growth. This means that smaller babies will be given a due date later than those measuring larger than the theory suggests. These are the babies that may have their due dates changed later in pregnancy or those who may be induced on the presumption that the baby is too large to birth and are at risk of shoulder dystocia (Wickham 2021). The message here seems to be that medical knowledge counts for more than a woman's own knowledge, yet nature cannot be predicted in such a fixed way. All birthing people and babies are individual. Pregnancy length varies because some babies need more time to grow and develop depending upon their individual genetic make-up. Therefore, the due date is an intervention that should be considered within the context of a date range and not a fixture on which to hang all other interventions, such as induction of labour. Of course, induction of labour has its place, especially when there is a significant medical need, such as placental insufficiency, foetal growth restriction or pre-eclampsia to name but a few, and when there is foetal or maternal compromise.

Another method of measurement and management occurs at the onset of labour in the form of routine vaginal examinations (NICE 2017) and labour progress plotted on a partogram or partograph. Put simply, the partogram is a paper graph where a woman's labour progress is plotted against a time frame with the intention of alerting midwives and obstetricians to take action when there is a deviation from normal expectations (Lavender, Cuthbert & Smyth 2018). Maternal observations such as blood pressure, pulse, temperature, urine output, contraction strength and length, and cervical dilatation plus foetal heart measurements are plotted on the graph to give a full overview of labour progress and foetal wellbeing. Beginning in the 1950s with Friedman (1954, 1955), followed by Philpott and Castle (1972), Studd (1973) and finally O'Driscoll, Stronge and Minogue (1973), cervical dilatation has been the measure by which to observe the 'ideal labour' (Downe & Byrom 2019). Just as all babies are expected to grow at the same rate, all women's cervixes are expected to open at the same rate as one another too – which most midwives will anecdotally tell you is preposterous. Women's bodies are unique and individual. When labour is spontaneous and physiology is in control, women's bodies will labour how they need to labour. Anecdotally, some women will labour quickly, some slowly; some women relax when they are in the hospital, some women labour more effectively at home; some women are responsive to their environment and labour can stop. Cervical dilatation is unpredictable, and yet according to the partogram, each woman in the active stage of labour (from 4cm dilated) is expected to labour pretty much like every other woman. Any deviation from the expectation of 1.2cm dilation per hour for primigravida women (those who have not given birth previously) and 1.5cm dilatation per hour for multiparous women (those who have given birth before) should be acted upon. There is no evidence so far that partogram use has contributed to improved maternal or foetal outcomes (Lavender *et al.* 2018; Lavender, Hart & Smyth 2008: Macdonald & Magill-Cuerden 2012; O'Connell, Martin & Dahlen 2022). Despite recommendations from the World Health Organization (WHO 2018), which advocate that cervical dilatation thresholds are unrealistic and that use of a partogram to identify women and babies at risk of adverse outcomes is not recommended, the partogram remains in use in the UK (NICE 2017).

The information presented here demonstrates how women's bodies have been categorised, routinised and forced into neat little boxes despite their bodies coming in all different shapes, sizes, ages, parity and genetic heredity. Women have differing menstrual cycle lengths and grow babies who require their own gestation period to grow, yet the imposed medical standards deem those bodies to be deficient and incompetent deviations from 'normal' because their actions do not fit within the neat little boxes (Macdonald & Magill-Cuerden 2012). From this view, medicalisation has impacted maternity practice pretty much the same as it has impacted the narratives around autism, especially in terms of the male-biased diagnostic tools used to diagnose and misdiagnose autistic women.

Whilst obstetric knowledge sits in the realm of medicine, science, categories, guidelines and algorithms, midwifery practice has one foot in this way of working and another foot in the *art* of midwifery. The very name midwife means 'with woman' (Kitzinger 1991), meaning that the midwife' remit is to walk alongside women during the perinatal period to support them in any way they need. Pregnancy, birth and the postnatal period are recognised as physiological processes which often need little intervention when left alone on their intended course. Women are supported on this journey with information which they can use to make informed choices and plan the care that is right for them. It is this experience that informs the art of midwifery practice. Midwives learn as much from women as the women learn from them in terms of observing the nuanced behaviours of women in labour to aid development of the embodied and intuitive knowledge discussed by Carper in 1978. Midwives do still work to the NICE guidelines and do still work within the realm of the medical model; however, there has been an increasing inclination towards a continuity-of-carer model with an emphasis on the midwife/mother relationship as central to improved outcomes for women and their babies (NHS England 2016).

Holistic and individualised care by the same midwife is beneficial for all women as they are less likely to experience preterm birth, pregnancy loss, episiotomies, use of regional analgesia and instrumental birth, and are more likely to receive streamlined postnatal and infant feeding support. Women report higher satisfaction with the information they receive and their ability to make informed choices about the place of birth and preparation for this, including being more likely to know the midwife if they wish to have a home birth (NHS England 2021). Women with low-risk pregnancies who choose to birth at home or in midwifery-led units are more likely to feel in control of their environment, especially in terms of sensory factors such as controlling the lighting, noise, items and people around them, and smells and tactile stimulation. Being in an environment of a woman's own choosing impacts movement, behaviour, responses, interactions, experience and stress levels. When women feel in control of the birth, their potential for a physiological undisturbed birth is maximised as stress hormones such as catecholamines are down-regulated, which enables oxytocin and endorphins, the hormones required for labour, to flow (Dooris & Rocca-Ihenacho 2019). Autistic women may find birthing in such environments with a known midwife reassuring, calming and empowering; however, choice is an important factor, and some people may find birthing under a consultant-led model with its restrictions and time limits more reassuring. For example, when women are given a 'due date', they follow a clearly defined plan of care (NICE 2021). Once the due date has been reached, women can have their labour induced or choose an elective caesarean section, so they have an almost guaranteed date on which to attend hospital. We say *almost* because nothing is certain in maternity care as we have already discussed, which can cause frustration when babies are not born on their due date or plans change. Of course, giving birth in a consultant-led unit may not be ideal for women with sensory differences. Such environments are loud, bright, disruptive and unpredictable, and so it is recommended that women are supported through individualised care to find the most appropriate care for them.

The information presented here demonstrates how midwifery care has struggled against male dominance of the priesthood together with male midwives, obstetricians and gynaecologists. Birth has moved from a social model into a medicalised one with the move of birth from home to hospital, then back again, with the recognition that mortality statistics were unmoved by the change. Birth is firmly placed in the technocratic paradigm whereby birth is a risky business that needs monitoring, measuring and managing, pretty much like all medical models seen within healthcare. The introduction of continuity of carer aims to redress the balance; however, at the time of writing, the continuity rollout has been paused due to unsafe staffing levels in the UK. This struggle back and forth between the models of maternity care is almost like a tug of war, and what needs to be recognised is the woman in the middle who stands with her determinants of health which require holistic, individualised care.

Current challenges in healthcare – pregnancy and birth

It seems that health services are under more pressure than ever before. The NHS is struggling to cope with unprecedented demand which exceeds capacity, a growing and ageing population, not enough qualified staff both due to demand and increasing recruitment and retention challenges, and the effects of the policy of austerity both within the NHS and upon the health of society as whole (Jones, Horton & Home 2022; Robertson *et al.* 2017).

Professional bodies have openly and increasingly shared concerns, with the BMA calling for an urgent meeting with the Prime Minister to discuss the crisis (Iacobucci 2017a, 2017b, 2017c, 2017d, 2017e), junior doctors taking strike action in the face of new contracts they feared did not provide 'robust contractual safeguards on safe working' (Rimmer 2018; see also Dyer 2016; Rimmer 2016; Roberts 2016; The Health Foundation 2016), and the advent and growth of the movement dubbed #saveournhs supported by the public and health professionals (Crane 2018; Ham 2017; King's Fund 2018; McCluskey 2017).

In times of such economic privation, the poorest, most vulnerable citizens are often the first to suffer (Sparrow 2015; Stubbs *et al.* 2022; Turner 2015). Specialist care practitioners and services such as those specialising in autism may be considered non-essential when faced with news reports of ambulance bays being reduced to parking lots, patients being left overnight on gurneys in hospital corridors and reports of crisis throughout the NHS (Campbell, Duncan & Marsh 2018; Evening Standard 2013; Glasby 2018; Ham 2017; Oliver 2018).

Current concerns in maternity care

Concerns about our healthcare system are shared by patients and professionals, with added stresses and strains of funding, training and staffing restrictions, increased bureaucracy which can lead to a reduction in flexibility and an unwillingness to admit where improvements can be made for fear of reprimand, seemingly in opposition to the principles of reflective practice, continuing professional development and patient-centred care. As Byrom and Downe (2015) state: 'Maybe the roar behind the silence is a roar of frustration at blinkered, blanket scientific-bureaucratic approaches, which do not respond passionately to the need for us to authentically engage with those who use our health services.'

There have been reports of a crisis in midwifery, with the RCM State of Maternity Services Report (2016) showing an ageing patient population and a rise in obesity, increasing risk of complications in the birthing process. The profession itself is ageing, with 35% of midwives in Wales being in their 50s and 60s, a pattern replicated across the UK, while current recruitment does not match demand. The RCM stated that 'more students need to be trained and brought into the health service as a matter of urgency', while they estimate a shortage of at least 3500 full-time midwives in England alone (RCM 2016). Scrapping the NHS bursary for student midwives and nurses in England correlated with a 23% drop in applicants (Jones-Berry 2017).

In the wider context of medicine, it's necessary to consider the effects of budgetary cuts and austerity measures in order to better contextualise why autistic birth may be under-served. For example, recent years have shown emerging concerns and public calls from NHS workers who believe patients' wellbeing and lives are being risked due to understaffing and lack of time to train effectively. Issues facing midwifery and mental health services have long been reported, yet the cases in media coverage are severe in nature, often featuring full-scale investigations into deaths. For example, local investigations into Prince Charles Hospital in Merthyr Tydfil reported that staff and budgetary shortages have directly impacted care, with often fatal consequences (Welsh Government 2019).

One could argue that superficial but sufficient 'awareness' training is relatively cost-effective, with few extra resources needed other than scheduled time for midwives to train. However, the current NHS working environment is under strict time/money constraints, which has meant the birth landscape has changed dramatically in recent years.

One of the forerunners of this change has been the Positive Birth Movement (PBM), founded by journalist and birth empowerment advocate Milli Hill. Central to the PBM movement, Hill believes birth isn't necessarily a medical event and that all power and consent should be put in the hands of the birthing mother. Hill's work builds upon that of Sheena Byrom, a consultant midwife who runs her own midwifery journal. Byrom uses lessons learned from the 1960s ethos of the medicalisation of birth to provide applicable changes in practice for modern-day issues.

The rise in PBM awareness has been paralleled by a recent rise in the use of doulas, who often take one of two roles: birth doula (prenatal and birth/labour help) and postnatal doula (postnatal help for parents to adjust to their new role at home).

As previously discussed, the NHS and midwifery units are reportedly under strain (De Benedictis & Gill 2016). Autism (and co-occurring conditions) awareness is increasing in medical and public sectors overall, but training can be inconsistent (Havercamp *et al.* 2016). Swansea Bay University Health Board, in line with other trusts across the UK, introduced an autism service under the title of 'Specialist Midwife in Learning Disability/Learning Difficulty/Hidden Disability/Autism' (Morgan 2019). In relation to the Better Births initiative (NHS England 2016), the roles were introduced with relevant training competencies. The learning objectives and robustness of the training is unknown, nor is it made explicit that autism awareness is required to be CPD (continuing professional development).

When considering the issues raised so far, from co-occurring issues to varied gender presentations, a robust approach is seemingly lacking when considering the complex issues so prevalent in the autistic population. One could argue that the mainstream medical knowledge of autism is inconsistent, particularly when viewing adult life events such as birth, or treating the autistic woman as an autonomous individual equal to her neurotypical peers.

Morgan (2019) found that autistic women negatively rated, or were not confident of, the knowledge of autism and related conditions of the medical professionals involved in birth preparation and birth experience.

- 'Q13 – I felt confident of the co-occurring conditions knowledge of medical professionals involved in birth preparation' – 51% could not agree.

- 'Q17 – I felt the medical professionals involved in the birth adequately understood my sensory needs' – 59.82% could not agree.

However, it is necessary to consider the effects of women answering retrospectively, with many reporting that they were undiagnosed at the time of birth. However, while medical professionals may not have been aware of the needs of the undiagnosed woman, the poor patient rating is arguably still relevant to any population regardless of diagnostic timing. As a result of this, while we want to find out the research related to the topic, we will be informed by the matters discussed thus far, such as the neurodiversity movement, disability stigma, PBM and autism awareness. This does not mean we won't be taking into account the work that doesn't meet these ideological standards, but it will inform how they are discussed. Additionally, mice studies, so common in autism research, will not be included: not only do they fail to represent the complex neurotype, but they aren't in poll position in the hierarchy of evidence either.

CHAPTER 2

Intersectionality and Feminism

This chapter will include research and statistics on the various intersections including other co-occurring conditions and disabilities, LGBTQIA+, and other issues more common in the autistic community (e.g. domestic abuse, bullying, sexual harassment). We will also include information from ethnic minorities, including the impact of cultural differences, underdiagnosis, stigma and stereotypes, as well as the findings of reports such as the MBRRACE report. Feminism will form a foundation here, with a retrospective investigation into the roots of gender disparity in healthcare.

- Overview
- Ethnic minorities
- LGBTQIA+
- Prior sexual trauma (re-emergence of prior trauma, re-emergence of childhood trauma/attachment issues/neglect upon becoming a new parent)
- Domestic violence
- Challenges in service provision
- Women's reproductive rights and the medicalisation of childbirth
- Over-medicalisation of childbirth and #MeToo in pregnancy and birth
- Obstetric violence
- PTSD-PC, mental health, PND and postpartum psychosis
- Stigma, judgement, emotional labour and fear of disclosure

- The autistic experience of breast/chestfeeding

Overview
Disparities in healthcare – specific challenges in healthcare and accessibility

- Diagnostic overshadowing

- Regular routine healthcare may be skipped or difficult (i.e. routine health checks, smears, dental, optician, etc.)

- Effects of medications/reactions

- Internalised ableism

- Communication problems

- Difficulties in maintaining sexual health and throughout pregnancy, birth and the postpartum period

- Lack of a holistic approach – services not integrating

Barriers to accessing adequate healthcare

- Telephone calls

- Speaking to the GP

- Short appointments

- Coping with examinations

- Coping with the waiting room and sensory environment

- Being perceived as rude or challenging when asking lots of questions

- Being perceived as overanxious, mentally ill or hypochondriac

- Keeping track of appointments, being on time

- Travel to and from appointments

- Being able to find, access, process, understand and respond to information

Autistic people 'as a group are heterogeneous, with a wide range of presentations, challenges and support needs', with limited or outdated understanding of the condition affecting healthcare providers' confidence and skill in catering to this section of the population (Doherty 2023).

The LeDeR Annual Report 2018 (Healthcare Quality Improvement Partnership 2019) showed huge negative discrepancies in healthcare and mortality.

Research has found that people with autism died over 16 years earlier than non-autistic people whilst another found that autistic adults with a learning disability died more than 30 years before non-autistic people (Croen *et al.* 2015; Hirvikoski *et al.* 2016; Mandell 2018; Nicolaidis *et al.* 2012), with a further study describing a twofold mortality risk for those with ASD (Schendel *et al.* 2016).

> I think a lot of care is needed to make sure the needs of people with ASD who are not able to communicate their views such as non-verbal people are not lost.
>
> I have experienced services that treat mental health and ASD as completely separate issues and both services seem fearful of people with the other condition. (Mind 2015, p.3)

Challenges in maintaining wellbeing for autistic/disabled people and how these may impact or be exacerbated by pregnancy, birth and adjusting to parenthood include:

- personal hygiene
- healthy diet
- regular exercise
- coping with isolation/difficulties accessing the community
- finances – difficulties with having enough money, a secure income or navigating the welfare system can make it difficult to afford appropriate housing, nutrition, social opportunities, etc. and affect our physical and mental health
- managing medications
- physical limitations on maintaining wellbeing such as being unable to chop food, stand for long periods, difficulty exercising, shopping and so on.

Impact of Covid-19 pandemic

This has had an impact on our health and wellbeing in many ways:

- Some of us may have had Covid-19, or have a family member who has.

- Others may have had routine or other healthcare appointments or procedures affected.

- Some people may be extremely nervous about attending the doctor, hospital or other appointments, or indeed even going out.

- Education, employment and finances may all have been affected, which can impact our physical and mental health.

- The ability to shop regularly may be impacted, which can affect health.

- For those with phobias around germs or compulsive hygiene routines, the pandemic may have been particularly difficult.

However, there have been positives – especially around accessibility. For example, there has been an increased facilitation of virtual appointments via Zoom/Skype, automated systems and other online healthcare portals. The pandemic has also facilitated – for some – better work/life balance, with more opportunities for blended learning, remote/flexible working and reduced travel burden, and with opportunities for community inclusion with online groups and events becoming more commonplace even as we progress into our 'new normal'.

Healthcare disparities – disability and disadvantage

There are many potential barriers to healthcare experienced by autistic people, which may include but are not limited to:

- sensory differences

- inaccessible systems/processes

- difficulty coping with clinical environments

- history of difficulty in healthcare/traumatic healthcare experiences

- limited self-advocacy skills

- intersectionality of disparities of gender, sexuality, race

- anxiety

- coexisting conditions/disabilities

- socioeconomic status

- travel considerations

- financial implications (particularly where free healthcare is not available)

- social difficulties

- communication differences

- perception of healthcare professionals (need for information, self-education, many conditions/health symptoms, lack of understanding, disbelief, etc.).

The impact of austerity on multiple disadvantage

Philip Alston, UN Special Rapporteur, reported in his preliminary findings from his visit to the UK in 2018:

> The costs of austerity have fallen disproportionately upon the poor, women, racial and ethnic minorities, children, single parents, and people with disabilities. The changes to taxes and benefits since 2010 have been highly regressive, and the policies have taken the biggest toll on those least able to bear it.

Austerity measures could be argued to be having a direct negative impact on health and maternity care, which we will explore below. However, austerity measures also have multiple impacts on disabled women across the World Health Organization's Wider Determinants of Health model, which suggests that people need, among other things, suitable employment, education, nutrition, housing, healthcare and community networks for overall wellbeing.

The UN Rapporteur Philip Alston noted that there was a substantial gender imbalance in the way austerity measures and welfare reform have been implemented in the UK, stating in a press conference, 'If you got a group of misogynists in a room and said "how can we make a system that works for men but not for women?", they wouldn't have come up with too many other ideas than what's in place' (Ward 2018).

Alston was damning in his report about how austerity disproportionately affects the vulnerable – women at risk of domestic violence, ethnic minority groups, the disabled (Alston 2018). The UN had already found the UK in breach of human rights on multiple occasions despite it being recorded as the fifth largest economy in the world (Butler 2017; Lambert 2017).

Recent research has shown that autistic students have lower rates of graduation and post-graduation employment than non-disabled students and students with other disabilities, with the exception of those with intellectual disabilities (Sarrett (2017), and have poorer outcomes in accessing housing (Churchard *et al.* 2018; Kargas *et al.* 2019) and affordable nutrition (May *et al.* 2019). They also experience compound difficulties with abusive relationships (Saxe 2017), in stress levels and mental health deterioration (Bates, Goodley & Runswick-Cole 2017), in stigma faced and subsequent impact on community inclusion and individual self-esteem (Burch 2017) and in an increase in perceived hostility in 'the system' which can include government agencies/departments, healthcare, local authorities, etc. leading to distrust, disillusionment and difficulties engaging with systems of care/support (McGrath, Griffin & Mundy 2016).

The impact of austerity measures on those facing multiple disadvantage can be catastrophic, with a report in the *BMJ* reporting 200,000 excess deaths in the UK – 100 per day – as a result of austerity (Watkins *et al.* 2017) and an author likening this to 'economic murder' in the press (Matthews-King 2017).

Gender: masking autistic characteristics and 'performing gender'

Women often 'camouflage' or 'mask' their autistic characteristics (Bargiela *et al.* 2016; Hull *et al.* 2017; Lai *et al.* 2015), which could further challenge clinicians in identifying and supporting this group. Autistic people often do not 'subscribe' to gender in conventional ways and may find additional difficulties in 'performing gender' in the loaded role of 'mother'. At the Autistica Discover Conference in 2019, it was commented that 'there is no more gendered position than that of "mother".'

Gender issues and intersectionality in autism diagnosis

Research has long reported the underdiagnosis of autism in women, often attributing this to issues such as gender bias in diagnostic tools and a resulting gender-specific awareness of the condition (Ratto *et al.* 2018). Seminal works on autism such as those on Theory of Mind and extreme male brain theory (Baron-Cohen 2002; Baron-Cohen *et al.* 1985) have been reported to further compound the underdiagnosis of women, when considering the higher frequency of social-seeking behaviours of autistic females. This has subsequently been linked to an underdiagnosis of autism in women, compounded by female 'masking' behaviours.

Standard deviation results for an autistic birth experience survey suggest that self-diagnosed and formally diagnosed women had statistically similar responses:

- SD self-identifying 1.376

- SD formal diagnosis 1.365.

(Morgan 2019)

The wider implications of this finding may impact care recommendations for the birth experience, as well as the validity of self-diagnosis of autism.

Wider research suggests that autism prevalence in the general population hasn't necessarily increased, with higher numbers being attributed to improved diagnostic efficacy (Wing & Potter 2002). With a rising number of diagnosed autistic women reaching adulthood, the medical and social support for such women have been considered absent or latent (Harmens, Sedgewick & Hobson 2022).

The concept of intersectionality is also gaining importance in midwifery and autism awareness (Ross 2018). This is described as a movement that seeks to bring prominence to the interconnected and overlapping nature of social categorisations such as race, social class, disability, gender and sexual orientation (Ross 2018). Intersectionality is particularly relevant to the higher prevalence of non-heteronormativity, underemployment and disability identity in the autistic community (George & Stokes 2017; Hayward, McVilly & Stokes 2018; Mogensen & Mason 2015).

Additionally, the female autistic population is more likely to have experienced sexual abuse, bullying and associated trauma (Schnabel & Bastow 2023). Along with masking and other complex coping mechanisms particular to autistic women, experiences specific to pregnancy and birth may be compounded by the alternative autistic pain experience – altered thresholds for hyper- and hyposensitivity (Baeza-Velasco et al. 2018).

> I was in pain and they said I was not even in labour. They were about to give me an epidural to shut me up despite my refusing it and struggling to get away from it when I said baby is crowning. They said rubbish. I said I would sue then they looked, and panic ensued as I was right. (Morgan 2019)

Historically, medical research has highlighted the importance of pain communication during pregnancy and birth with regard to the safety of mother and baby (Labor & Maguire 2008). Given these issues, it is fair to say that the experience of pregnancy and birth has the potential to affect autistic women in ways distinct from their neurotypical peers. The current literature based on autistic birth research is heavily reliant on reports from medical professionals and social workers. Some research has found that core symptoms such as social interaction 'deficits' and rigidity (of thought, verbal and body language) can put the autistic patient at a disadvantage during medical care appointments (McDonnell & DeLucia 2021).

In terms of gender and sexuality, autistic women are 30 times more likely to be non-heterosexual (George & Stokes 2017) and gender non-conforming. As already mentioned, this may impact dysphoria or trauma-related issues.

Ethnic minorities

Cultural differences make a huge difference to the personal experience of pregnancy and childbirth. Whether this is in the likelihood to access adequate support, respect of self-advocacy or even pain reporting, an autistic person from an ethnic minority will face even more inherent biases and injustices during their journey to parenthood.

This is further confounded for those from ethnic minorities and those of lower socioeconomic background, who access fewer services from diagnosis throughout the lifespan (Begeer *et al.* 2009).

The increasing awareness of intersectionality in person-centred antenatal care has also seen prominent doulas such as Mars Lord educate professionals about the importance of intersectionality, as a result of the MBRRACE report (2021) that states that Black women are five times more likely to die in childbirth; data also suggest that disabled women also face more complications giving birth (Mitra *et al.* 2015). The importance of intersectionality – namely differences in gender, sexuality, race and learning difficulties – is key to understanding the bigger picture of where research on the autistic birth experience fits.

More specifically, the barriers an autistic person from an ethnic minority background may face giving birth may be more extensive than for a white autistic person. For example, Black women often face stigma from their behaviour being interpreted as more aggressive or their pain levels disbelieved (Bamber *et al.* 2023), which is anecdotally echoed in the autistic community.

LGBTQIA+

Autistic people are 34 times more likely to be non-heterosexual than their neurotypical counterparts. While research is beginning to embrace late identification of non-heterosexual identity of parents, there is little available research focusing specifically on the intersectionality of autism and sexual identity minorities. With the higher likelihood that the autistic pregnant person will have a different experience in this sense, it is worth being aware of this fact when aiming to support pregnant autistic people and their partners.

Prior sexual trauma (re-emergence of prior trauma, re-emergence of childhood trauma/attachment issues/neglect upon becoming a new parent)

Prior sexual trauma was identified as the most prominent risk factor for PTSD in women following childbirth (Verreault *et al.* 2012). Women often experience profound subconscious effects whilst navigating a potentially painful labour involving those body parts affected by prior abuse (Gottfried *et al.* 2015; Güneş & Karaçam 2017; Roberts *et al.* 2023). Although midwives should be mindful of prior trauma, the intense pressure they face can reduce the time available to each patient, alongside the possibility that prior trauma may not be disclosed, which may potentially impact care (Koblinsky *et al.* 2016).

There is an increased incidence of sexual abuse among autistic women, and in women with the commonly co-occurring condition ADHD, which can make this a heightened consideration (Brown-Lavoie, Viecili & Weiss 2014; Eberjer *et al.* 2012; Ohlsson Gotby *et al.* 2018).

Domestic violence

- Over a third of domestic violence starts or becomes worse when a woman is pregnant.

- 15% of women report violence during their pregnancy.

- 40–60% of women experiencing domestic violence are abused while pregnant.

- More than 14% of maternal deaths occur in women who have told their health professional they are in an abusive relationship.

(Home Office 2023; Oppenheim 2021)

Domestic violence is a heightened concern for women in pregnancy. Autistic women are more likely to have a lack of social support or perceived social support and to enter into and stay longer in abusive relationships (Bargiela *et al.* 2016; Maddox & White 2015). Disabled women are not only more likely to experience physical abuse, but they are also more likely to experience it during pregnancy (Mitra, Manning & Lu 2012).

Healthcare disparity is an area in which autistic women are likely to be facing multiple barriers – due to both autism and being female (Mitchell & Schlesinger 2005). This can be further compounded by the intersectionality of other factors.

It seems that this disparity is pronounced enough to contribute to poorer health – physical and mental – with a likelihood of multiple chronic conditions and a substantial increase in mortality rates for autistic people, with these rates suggested to be as much as double those of the non-ASD population, and spanning almost all causes of death (Croen *et al.* 2015; Hirvikoski *et al.* 2016; Nicolaidis *et al.* 2014; Nicolaidis & Raymaker 2013; Preißmann 2017; Schendel *et al.* 2016).

While some issues are systemic/environmental, or related to communication differences or difficulties in self-advocacy, others can be related to professionals having limited or outdated understanding of autism which affects their confidence and skill in catering to this section of the population (Nicolaidis *et al.* 2012).

Where an autistic person has a learning disability, this can compound disparities further, with the 2018 and 2019 Learning Disabilities and Mortality Reviews (Healthcare Quality Improvement Partnership 2019, 2020) showing significant disparities in health and mortality, even reporting that up to 19 do-not-resuscitate orders (DNRs) were signed between 2016 and 2018 where LD/ID or Down's syndrome was reported as justification for this.

There have been tragic instances of autistic people losing their lives in health and social care systems, including Oliver McGowan, who was prescribed an antipsychotic against his wishes and the wishes of his parents, leading to a catastrophic reaction; Connor Sparrowhawk, who was epileptic and died after being left unsupervised in a bathtub; and Richard Handley, who suffered extreme faecal impaction (BBC 2019; Halliday 2018; Handley 2016).

Perhaps the most tragic aspect of Richard Handley's death was that a woman died in similar circumstances a mere six months later, leading his sister to question whether 'timely investigation and service improvements' could have changed this outcome (Handley 2016).

This disparity extends not only to medical care but also social care systems, with instances of disadvantage including actual abuse being suffered by those who are autistic and/or have an LD, such as the Winterbourne and Whorlton Hall scandals (Mitchell 2019; The Health Foundation 2019) or, on a much more widely reported scale, autistic people being kept in secure units for lengthy amounts of time, past suggested guidelines or far away from their homes and families due to a lack of sufficient appropriate social care environments.

The issues faced can lead to disillusion and distrust of the healthcare system (Bargiela *et al.* 2016), which could add another layer of difficulty to engaging with and treating autistic patients. This perhaps accounts for the decline in autistic people accessing healthcare with age (Nathenson & Zablotsky 2017), and findings suggesting autistic adults may be more disadvantaged than children, with professionals reporting less understanding of how autism presents in adults (Croen *et al.* 2015).

Specific to women's reproductive health, research suggests autistic women are less likely to access gynaecological care (Zerbo *et al.* 2019). Accounts also suggest that disabled women may be unable to access routine smears even when they attempt to (Jo's Blog 2019).

Lum, Garnett and O'Connor (2014) found that autistic women suffered greater anxiety and distress generally in accessing healthcare due to difficulties in communication, sensory issues and social anxiety, further finding that these difficulties meant they faced increased stress in childbirth, often with difficulties in reporting pain levels or in feeling supported and informed.

Morgan (2019) found that the impact of the medical environment compounded by an autistic tendency to experience sensory overwhelm was illustrated, with patients reporting a negative rating of 37.74% (strongly disagree and slightly disagree) agreeing with the statement 'I felt my sensory needs were considered seriously at the appointments'. This may be influential on the similarly negative response (34.54% strongly disagree and slightly disagree) for 'I felt like I could communicate my needs effectively to the midwife'. This finding suggests that appointment environments are failing to help facilitate fundamental communication.

It can be argued that our healthcare system has a tradition of being patriarchal or even misogynistic in nature, from its history of 'hysterical women' to its modern-day dismissal of women's concerns, with female pain often being treated differently to that of males (Samulowitz *et al.* 2018; Williams & Mann 2017).

Studies show that autistic people are more likely to belong to the LGBTQIA+ community and that this group is also likely to face barriers and stigma in healthcare (Cooper, Smith & Russell 2018; George & Stokes 2017; Glidden *et al.* 2016; Øien, Cicchetti & Nordahl-Hansen 2018; Somerville 2015; Stewart & O'Reilly 2017). With emerging research suggesting that autistic people are more likely to have gender identity differences, whether that be trans, non-binary or other preferred identity, there are issues around understanding, treatment and postnatal care including chestfeeding for this group (MacDonald *et al.* 2016).

Those from ethnic minority backgrounds also experience barriers in healthcare, both generally and specifically to maternity care (Garcia *et al.* 2015). The National Perinatal Epidemiology Unit (NPEU) MBRRACE-UK reports (MBRRACE-UK 2018a, 2018b) showed shocking disparities in deaths of Black and Asian women compared to their white counterparts, as well as disparities in survival rates of their infants.

According to the 2018 MBRRACE-UK report *Saving Lives, Improving Mothers' Care*, 'In 2014–2016. 9.8 per 100,000 women died during pregnancy or up to six weeks after childbirth or the end of pregnancy. Most women who died had multiple health problems or other vulnerabilities' (MBRRACE-UK 2018a). These findings are stark, and while the report doesn't take disability into account as a variable, given how strongly other research suggests that autistic people are more likely to have both a higher number of health conditions and vulnerability, arguably this provides essential context for how much more vulnerable autistic women are in pregnancy and postnatal timeframes.

'Black women are five times more likely…to die [in pregnancy] compared to white women' (MBRRACE-UK 2018a). As white women, we cannot and will not speak on the behalf of Black women or replace their voices, but we feel it is our basic human duty to point out the tragedy, injustice and multiple levels of prejudice Black autistic women will face during the transition to parenthood. We strongly believe that the intersectionality between disability/autism and parenthood needs serious investment for publishers, and engagement from the general public and health professionals alike. Just as racism is a systemic injustice, tackling the issue for disabled parents from ethnic minorities requires at least equally weighted change. We urge everyone reading this book to take on the emotional labour of educating themselves about this topic, putting in the work to make change and elevating the voices of parents from ethnic minority backgrounds.

While we are aware that small sections of this book are insufficient to address the topic of intersectionality from the patient voice, we urge readers to follow the blogs, social media accounts and other events geared specifically to listening to experiences of those from ethnic minority backgrounds in this part of the lifespan. Examples include:

- @Mis_Taught (Twitter)/@mistaught.uk (Instagram) aka Melissa, an autism educator and champion of rights for autistic people from ethnic minority backgrounds

- @chineseautismuk (Twitter), headed by Hazel Lim, which aims to 'empower parents and advocate for Chinese families living with autism; promote understanding of autism within Chinese community against the strong stigma'

- @MorenikeGO (Twitter) – Morénike Giwa Onaiwu, 'Mom, writer, disability justice/race/gender/anti-HIV stigma advocate; survivor #Neurodivergent AuDHD enby woman w/alopecia and mild young-onset dementia'

- @BobbVenessa (Twitter) – Venessa Swaby (Bobb), 'My journey, my interests and other issues I have experienced, that need to be addressed. Autism, Abuse, Exploitation, Young Mums, My Faith'

- @BlackAutistics (Twitter) – Black Autistics 'Researching Autism at the intersection of Racial, Ethnic, Cultural and Socioeconomic Diversity'.

Despite the evidence that clearly shows the barriers for these groups, stigma persists, still tending to place the 'blame' squarely on those being failed by the system, suggesting it is due to factors such as differences in genetics, body type, lifestyle choice and poor socioeconomic background (Gibert, DeGrazia & Danis 2017; Macias 2018).

Our healthcare system is under immense pressure in its entirety and for the individual professionals working within it, and although we claim to value evidence-based and continued professional development and reflective practice, we seem to have fostered a culture where it is so terrifying to make a mistake – or even worse admit to one – that instead we have professionals 'playing it safe', afraid to offer options and extend their practice, and to be transparent in their failings. These are clearly areas in need of improvement to grow both individually and as a collective professional group (Lyndon *et al.* 2015). This often means that maternity care choices are restricted, narrow pathways of care are followed, examinations are strongly recommended and interventions happen too early and too often (Kay 2019; Lokugamage & Pathberiya 2017). When coupled with some healthcare providers admitting to being unprepared to deal with autistic patients – with 77% in one study rating their ability to do so as poor or fair – there is reason for substantial concern (Croen *et al.* 2015; Zerbo *et al.* 2015).

Challenges in service provision

It seems that health services are under more pressure than ever before. The NHS is struggling to cope with unprecedented demand which exceeds capacity, a growing and ageing population, not enough qualified staff both due to demand and increasing recruitment and retention challenges, and the effects of austerity both within the NHS and upon the health of society as whole (Jones *et al.* 2022; Robertson *et al.* 2017).

Professional bodies have openly and increasingly shared concerns, with the BMA calling for an urgent meeting with the Prime Minister to discuss the crisis (Iacobucci 2017a, 2017b, 2017c, 2017d, 2017e), junior doctors taking strike action in the face of new contracts they feared did not provide 'robust contractual safeguards on safe working' (Dyer 2016; Rimmer 2016, 2018), and the advent and growth of the movement dubbed #saveournhs supported by the public and health professionals (Ham 2017; King's Fund 2018; McCluskey 2017).

There have been reports of a crisis in midwifery, with the RCM State of Maternity Services Report (2016) showing an ageing patient population and a rise in obesity increasing risk of complications in the birthing process. The profession itself is ageing, with 35% of midwives in Wales being in their 50s and 60s, a pattern replicated across the UK, whilst current recruitment does not match demand. The RCM stated that 'more students need to be trained and brought into the health service as a matter of urgency', whilst they estimate a shortage of at least 3500 full-time midwives in England alone (RCM 2016). Scrapping the NHS bursary for student midwives and nurses has correlated with a 23% drop in applicants (Jones-Berry 2017).

In times of such economic privation, the poorest, most vulnerable citizens are often the first to suffer (Rickard Straus & Barrow 2013; Sparrow 2015; Turner 2015). Specialist care practitioners and services such as those specialising in autism may be considered non-essential when faced with news reports of ambulance bays being reduced to parking lots, patients being left overnight on gurneys in hospital corridors and reports of crisis throughout the NHS (Donnelly 2015; Ham 2017; Campbell, Duncan & Marsh 2018; Oliver 2018; Glasby 2018).

Despite this, services must provide the best care possible, and legislation means equality cannot be overlooked. The Autism Act 2009 in England states that there must be an autism strategy which provides guidance to the NHS, including planning of relevant services for autistic adults and training of staff who provide these services. Legal implications for failures under such legislation – along with the Equality Act 2010, Human Rights Act 1998, UN Convention on the Rights of Persons with Disabilities 2006 or the Disability Discrimination Act 2005 – can potentially lead to litigation with negative financial implications. Thus, the temptation to save money in the short term on specialist care may prove to be short-sighted in the long run.

Autistic people are more likely to face disparity in healthcare, with limited or outdated understanding of the condition affecting healthcare providers' confidence and skill in catering to this section of the population (Nicolaidis *et al.* 2012). Difficulties with communication and social interaction can further compound this issue, leading to widespread impairment in self-advocacy. The LeDeR report (Healthcare Quality Improvement Partnership 2019) showed huge negative discrepancies in healthcare and mortality in those with LD, while Hirvikoski *et al.* (2016) and Mandell (2018) made similar findings specific to autism, with Schendel *et al.* (2016) describing a twofold mortality risk for those with ASD.

Autistic women were shown to be significantly less likely to access gynaecological care by Zerbo *et al.* (2018), while Lum, Garnett and O'Connor (2014) found that autistic women suffered greater anxiety and distress generally in accessing healthcare due to difficulties in communication, sensory issues and social anxieties, further finding that these difficulties meant they faced increased stress in childbirth, often with difficulties in reporting pain levels or in feeling supported and informed. Both studies were conducted overseas, in America and Australia respectively, so studies in the UK would be beneficial to see if similar barriers are faced here.

Healthcare providers in the US admitted to being unprepared to deal with autistic patients, with 77% rating their ability to do so as poor or fair, and showing a general lack of awareness of how many autistic patients may be in their care – with only 2% of providers in a study reporting more than ten autistic adults in their care when half of providers were treating this number (Croen *et al.* 2015; Zerbo *et al.* 2015). Croen *et al.* (2015) further found autistic adults may be at even more of a disadvantage than children, with professionals reporting less understanding of how autism presents in adults, also finding 25% of professionals wished to improve this. It seems possible barriers such as time and funding may be hindering progress. Again, although data from such a large-scale study is valuable, UK-based studies would be warranted to see if such trends remain applicable here.

This disparity in healthcare may be increased when consideration is given to the finding that autistic people are more likely to fit into other marginalised groups. For example, the rate of autistic people in the LGBTQ community has increased (Cooper *et al.* 2018; George & Stokes 2017; Øien *et al.* 2018), a group also known to face differing needs and disparity in healthcare and stigma (Glidden *et al.* 2016; Somerville 2015; Stewart & O'Reilly 2017). Women also face disparity in healthcare, often with their pain being treated differently to that of males (Samulowitz *et al.* 2018; Williams & Mann 2017).

Autistic people are more likely to suffer socioeconomic deprivation. When you consider the wider determinants of health, these are often negatively affected in the ASD population. Education is often negatively impacted, with many individuals facing difficulties or breakdown in accessing education (NAS 2021a). Autistic adults are less likely to be in employment, particularly full-time employment, as are their carers (Carers UK 2014). This has a snowball effect on financial circumstances, housing, nutrition and community engagement, and may therefore also impact the birth process because of stigma or difficulties with self-advocacy due to lack of education or low self-esteem.

Carers such as a family member or spouse may be able to mitigate these issues in some circumstances; however, autistic women are less likely to have a strong social support network (Maddox & White 2015) and are more likely to suffer abuse (Bargiela *et al.* 2016). Women with disabilities are not only more likely to suffer physical abuse, but they are also more likely to suffer it during pregnancy (Mitra *et al.* 2012).

There is an increased incidence of sexual abuse shown in autistic women, albeit in Canadian and Swedish studies (Brown-Lavoie *et al.* 2014; Ohlsson Gotby *et al.* 2018), which further complicates the patient profile. Ohlsson Gotby *et al.* (2018) conducted a large-scale study on 4500 participants which is extremely valuable; however, they did experience a significant non-response rate which may influence their findings.

Increased risk is also associated with the common comorbidity of ADHD (Eberjer *et al.* 2012).

Impairments in executive functioning and central coherence mean that a different environment and unpredictable and unfamiliar chain of events can be almost impossible to deal with, particularly when the added difficulty of emotional regulation is considered (Kiep & Spek 2017; Lemon *et al.* 2011; Mazefsky *et al.* 2013).

Autistic women may appear difficult, uncooperative or spoiled to busy staff when actually they are overwhelmed, on the verge of or fully immersed in fight, flight or freeze mode. It is important to show compassion and patience rather than dismissing these difficulties, although without some understanding of the root cause of this outward behaviour, midwives may find this difficult.

Autistic women are often shown to 'camouflage' or 'mask' their traits (Bargiela *et al.* 2016; Hull *et al.* 2017; Lai *et al.* 2015), which could further confuse clinicians in identifying and supporting this group. All studies cited here focused solely on women they classed as high-functioning (i.e. without any intellectual disability). Therefore, this may not generalise across the spectrum. Bargiela *et al.* (2016) conducted a qualitative study that focused on only 14 participants, which provided depth to the findings, but this research would need to be expanded to see if the results replicate across a larger section of the population.

These factors suggest a real risk of trauma during the birth process, both to the expectant mother and her partner (Iles, Slade & Spiby 2011; Inglis, Sharman & Reed 2016). Interestingly, research suggests that the perception of danger and trauma is just as important as clinically observable physical danger, with many women affected experiencing uncomplicated vaginal births (Söderquist, Wijma & Wijma 2006).

Autistic individuals are more likely to experience PTSD (Roberts *et al.* 2015). Research shows that those who suffer from anxiety, those with a history of sexual abuse or domestic violence, and those with a poor support network are more likely to experience PTSD (Verrault *et al.* 2012). As we have discussed, autistic women are more likely to fall into these categories, which increases their risk.

The impact of such trauma can be profound and far-reaching. It can lead to postnatal depression (PND) and depression in women and their partners, which can in turn impact infant bonding and wellbeing (Iles *et al.* 2011; Inglis *et al.* 2016).

Mitra *et al.* (2015) found that there were increased complications in pregnancy and birth in women with intellectual and developmental disabilities (IDDs). However, these studies, although large-scale, were conducted in the US and were not autism-specific.

Unfortunately, much of the evidence discussed here is small-scale and limited in scope. A lot of the papers focused on those termed high-functioning, a trend that has been noted in research, which is far from ideal as up to 70% of autistic people have an accompanying intellectual disability (ID) (Matson & Cervantes 2014). Most of the content is not specific to maternity care, and much of the theoretical basis, such as that relating to genetic differences in pain, is very much in its infancy. There is a crucial need for evidence across all discussed factors to be drawn together cohesively and focused on the autistic population, with real community engagement, to fully understand the experiences and difficulties faced, thus informing future best practice.

Women's reproductive rights and the medicalisation of childbirth

In the words of Bashi Hazard, a lawyer and board member of Human Rights in Childbirth, a birth plan 'is the closest expression of informed consent that a woman can offer her caregiver prior to commencing labour' (Hill 2019a).

Despite this assertion, it seems that many women have birth plans dismissed, denied or overlooked during the birth process. The following statistics are from an online survey conducted by the Positive Birth Movement and Channel Mum (2016):

- 75% made a birth plan.

- Only half of those birth plans were read by professionals.

- 42% said their plan was not adhered to.

There even seems to be a prevailing attitude that women who create birth plans are hippy, pushy, unrealistic, entitled females to be mocked and ridiculed for their expression of their wishes, as described in Adam Kay's book *This Is Going to Hurt*, in much in the same vein as an online blog post by a self-proclaimed 'satirical medical news website', allegedly run by 'stressed healthcare professionals' (Gomer Blog 2014) and in a Twitter exchange between obstetricians that 'joked' that 'the length of the birth plan directly correlates to the length of the caesarean incision' and 'laminated birth plans were only useful if the woman had a massive haemorrhage' (Hill 2019a).

Patient HJ needs an emergency caesarean section for failure to progress in labour. This has not come as a surprise. When I met her on admission, she presented me with her nine-page birth plan, in full colour and laminated. The whale song that would be playing on her laptop (I don't remember the exact breed of whale but I'm pretty sure it was documented to that level of detail), the aromatherapy oils that would be used, and introduction to the hypnotherapy techniques she would be employing, a request for the midwife to say 'surges' rather than 'contractions'. The whole thing was doomed from the start – having a birth plan always strikes me as akin to having a 'what I want the weather to be' plan or a 'winning the lottery' plan. (Kay 2018)

When asked about writing a birth plan, only 14.85% of respondents (Morgan 2019) agreed that they wrote the plan collaboratively with medical professionals involved in their birth. For context, a birth plan may be considered a very personal document or something that a birthing mother could write with their partner. While, as a discrete statistic, this number may reflect these matters, when in context of other poor ratings around autonomy and accommodations, there is cause for concern here. For example, only 27.7% of women agreed with the statement 'I felt generally well-informed of what was going on during birth'. While certain aspects of birth may often evoke feelings of powerlessness for many women, when coupled with other results related to consent and bodily autonomy, it could be argued that autistic women experience informed consent practices poorly.

Two centuries of obstetricians have found no way of predicting the course of a labour, but a certain denomination of floaty-dressed mother seems to think she can manage it easily.

Adam Kay, *This is Going to Hurt* (2018)

It seems no woman is exempt from scrutiny and disdain over her birth choices – Meghan Markle, Duchess of Sussex, was criticised for wearing high heels in pregnancy and her reported wish to have a home birth (Dear 2019; Schiller 2019). This is a societal issue that reinforces the belief that women's choices are frivolous, unimportant, ridiculous, and that women are 'spoilt' for believing they have a right to a voice in the process.

Morgan (2019) found that autistic women struggle to have their voice heard in birth. Most notably, only 14.05% of respondents could agree with the statement 'I felt confident in communicating my emotions during birth'. Furthermore, the resulting lack of voice had a negative impact on needs being met by accommodations in practice, with only 8.43% of respondents agreeing with the statement 'The ward made adequate accessibility adjustments for me'.

Over-medicalisation of childbirth and #MeToo in pregnancy and birth

Hill (2019a) states that birth is a feminist issue, and in the landscape of the global #MeToo movement, consent in childbirth is a matter of long-overdue debate. Many women feel overruled, disempowered or violated in the birth process, with these words commonly occurring throughout the literature along with words such as silent, unheard, damaged, cornered, disposable, overridden, unimportant, degraded, coerced, endured, infantilised, overwhelmed. The list goes on but the picture it paints is a disheartening one.

At a policy level, the NICE guidelines for 'Complicated Pregnancy' (NICE 2019) have noticeably fewer options focused on maternal autonomy and decision making, while the 'Uncomplicated Pregnancy' guidelines have a lot more options of this kind (NICE 2021). This may illustrate how the autistic birth experience may face policy-level issues from fundamental differences in service design and guideline impact before midwife autism awareness training is factored.

Medical professionals, including midwives, reported a reciprocated difficulty with interacting with autistic mother patients (Suplee *et al.* 2014). For example, Suplee and colleagues (2014) also found that the autistic mother's body language was interpreted as defensive, tone of voice was difficult to gauge intention from and direct manners were gauged as hostile despite true intentions. Furthermore, primary care physicians have self-reported low confidence and inadequate skills when caring for autistic people (Parellada *et al.* 2013). This may suggest that service-level as well as interpersonal barriers exist in many dimensions for autistic adults accessing healthcare, as the following statistics from the Birthrights Dignity in Childbirth Survey illustrate (Birthrights 2013).

- Only 68% of women were given a choice of where to give birth.

- 31% said they did not feel in control of their birth experience.

- 15% were unhappy with the availability of pain relief and 10% were unhappy with the choice of pain relief.

- 23% were unhappy about not being given a choice of position during labour.

- 20% said healthcare professionals did not always introduce themselves.

- 18% did not feel that health professionals listened to them.

- 12% did not consider that they had consented to medical procedures.

- 24% of women who had an instrumental birth said they had not consented to procedures.

The World Health Organization has advocated for empowerment of women in labour, with the publication of their guidance for intrapartum care (WHO 2018), quoted below, followed by the list of principles:

> The growing knowledge on how to initiate, accelerate, terminate, regulate, or monitor the physiological process of labour and childbirth has led to an increasing medicalisation of the process. It is now being understood that this approach may undermine a woman's own capability in giving birth and could negatively impact her experience of what should normally be a positive, life-changing experience.

The guidance proposes 'care throughout labour and birth including essential physical resources and competent and motivated staff' with these key guidelines:

- Respectful labour and childbirth care: Respectful maternity care – which refers to care organised for and provided to all women in a manner that maintains their dignity, privacy and confidentiality, ensures freedom from harm and mistreatment, and enables informed choice and continuous support during labour and childbirth – is recommended.

- Emotional support from a companion of choice: A companion of choice is recommended for all women throughout labour and childbirth.

- Effective communication by staff: Effective communication between maternity care providers and women in labour, using simple and culturally acceptable methods, is recommended.

- Continuity of care: Midwife-led continuity-of-care models, in which a known midwife or small group of known midwives supports a woman throughout the antenatal, intrapartum and postnatal continuum, are recommended for pregnant women in settings with well-functioning midwifery programmes.

- Pre-established referral plan.

- Pain relief strategies.

- Oral fluid and food intake.

- Regular labour monitoring, documentation of events, audit and feedback.

- Mobility in labour and birth position of choice.

(WHO 2018)

Obstetric violence

The emergence of a new term 'obstetric violence', originating in Venezuela, is defined as:

> The appropriation of a woman's body and reproductive processes by health personnel, in the form of dehumanising treatment, abusive medicalization and pathologization of natural processes, involving a woman's loss of autonomy and of the capacity to freely make her own decisions about her body and sexuality, which has negative consequences for a woman's quality of life. (Sadler *et al.* 2016, cited in Nagle & Samari 2021)

The following list, from Venezuelan law, of what constitutes obstetric violence is also helpful. It encompasses (Pérez D'Gregorio 2010):

- untimely and ineffective attention to obstetric emergencies

- forcing the woman to give birth in a supine position when the necessary means to perform a vertical delivery are available

- impeding early attachment of the child with his/her mother without a medical cause

- altering the natural process of low-risk labour and birth by using augmentation techniques

- performing caesarean sections when natural childbirth is possible, without obtaining the voluntary, expressed and informed consent of the woman.

Both action and inaction can be violent, and violating. Neglecting a woman in labour who is asking for pain relief or stating that something is wrong, denying access to a caesarean or intervening too late could be considered acts of violence, just as the 'too much too soon' approach can also be violent, undermining a woman's autonomy and depriving her of the chance to experience her own bodily capabilities. (Hill 2019b)

The coining of the term 'obstetric violence' and its enshrining in Venezuelan law may be a pathway the rest of the world is likely to follow, particularly in the West where concerns have been raised about too much intervention, too soon, and the 'over-medicalisation of childbirth' (WHO 2018).

PTSD-PC, mental health, PND and postpartum psychosis

PTSD-PC and mental health issues such as anxiety, postnatal depression and, in extreme cases, postpartum psychosis have been highlighted as a concern (Iles *et al.* 2011; Inglis *et al.* 2016; Maternal Mental Health Alliance 2018).

Morgan (2019) found that 40.95% of respondents reported they had lacked autonomy over being touched by medical professionals when responding to the statement 'I felt I had consent about how and when I was touched during observations'. For a population more likely to have suffered trauma, abuse and gender dysmorphic traits, autistic women arguably require more opportunities for consent and bodily autonomy. On a practical, service-level, responses included:

- 'I knew where to access support after appointments' – 45.37% could not agree they were informed.

- 'I knew how to inform the medical practice if I was not happy with my care' – 51.39% could not agree they were informed.

- 'I knew I had the right to change midwives if I needed to' – 49.79% could not agree they were informed.

Overall, this suggests that during early pregnancy care, autistic women are at a disadvantage on service, delivery and interpersonal levels.

Traumatic birth can leave a huge impact on women and their families, with research showing it is the perception of trauma that is important, even if 'on paper' a birth seems uncomplicated (Söderquist *et al.* 2006). Indeed, in births where complications or interventions were necessary, it was not the actual interventions that were the cause of trauma but the 'interactions around' interventions (Hollander *et al.* 2017).

A study by Verrault *et al.* (2012) identified risk factors for development of PTSD-PC, including a lack of perceived social support, a history of sexual trauma, higher anxiety, sensitivity and a more negative childbirth experience than expected, all of which are arguably more likely to exist in autistic people (Bargiela *et al.* 2016; Brown-Lavoie *et al.* 2014; Maddox & White 2015; McGonigle *et al.* 2014).

Partners/fathers are also at risk of tokophobia, PTSD-PC or depression in the postpartum period, particularly if the birth was perceived as traumatic and/or their partner developed these conditions (Bradley & Slade 2011; Ganapathy 2015; Iles *et al.* 2011). Many fathers reported feeling helpless, uninformed and frustrated during birth, which can have significant impact (Inglis *et al.* 2016).

Stigma, judgement, emotional labour and fear of disclosure

Autistic parents – and expectant parents – are often afraid of disclosing their diagnosis and needs, of being vulnerable in a system that has often failed us (Hill 2017). This is reinforced by the negative messages that continually appear in the media and from society – in the past couple of years alone, we have faced the storm of #puppetgate, an extremely problematic play whereby the autistic character was portrayed by a puppet alongside an all-human cast, a play about autistic mothers that caused outrage, and overwhelming attacks on the young autistic climate-change campaigner Greta Thunberg that seem to fixate on her age, gender and neurotype (Jones 2019; Ryan 2019).

In literature and the press, there has been further stigma – a book by a mother of an autistic child that was widely criticised, and a Harvard psychologist who has created advice around 'mixed-neurotype' relationships which suggests neurotypical partners of autistic people are at risk of abuse, further suggesting neurotypical parents are always better placed to care for children than autistic parents (Cassidy 2019). This is perpetuated by harmful media campaigns by organisations such as Autism Speaks (ASAN 2009; Bever 2019), and we are even seeing parents administering bleach enemas to their autistic children in hopes of a 'cure' (Burstow 2019).

In echoes of the days of 'refrigerator mothers', autistic parents are often judged for their differences, assumed to be incapable or fundamentally misunderstood, with allegations of FII a concern (Pohl *et al.* 2016). This is well illustrated in the two quotes below.

> But part of me is glad that I didn't know I was autistic until I already had children. I don't know that I would have been brave enough to have had them, had I known I was autistic. I might well have been too cautious to think I could be a good mother. I only admit I'm autistic to better support my daughters and jump hurdles on their behalf. There is so much judgement against autistic mothers that I consider myself genuinely lucky never to have been subjected to the interrogation of the social service professionals. It's a constant cause of terror for autistic mothers. (Hill 2017)

> I've never seen a shirt saying Autistic and Pregnant or something along those lines. Probably because it wouldn't be safe to wear. It hurts. It hurts that it's not safe to wear a shirt like that. It hurts remembering the signs at pro-choice rallies, saying that 'an autistic woman shouldn't be forced to give birth' as if autism has anything to do with the fact that no-one should be forced to be pregnant and ignoring the fact that an autistic woman shouldn't be forced to abort, either. It hurts to know that people legitimately think that Autistic people either can't or shouldn't have kids. Can't would be the assumption that Autistic people wouldn't be able to. We can. We do. Why do you think we still exist? People like us can grow up and have kids. It's not just broad autism phenotypers who have autistic kids. It's autistic adults who have autistic kids too. (Hillary 2013)

> When one's pregnant and makes it known you do have to expect some degree of unsolicited advice from others. What I didn't expect was the mass amounts of ableist hate I'd get thrown at me…even by parents of autistic children. 'If you're autistic why did you get pregnant?' 'How could you do that to a child?' 'You're just going to have an autistic kid! How are you really going to handle that when you have problems?' 'You really have no business having kids' and other such malarkey. (Autistic People Speaking Out 2013)

Groups and communities both online and locally can be difficult for autistic parents to engage in; increasingly, there is a struggle for power and dominance of the narrative around autism which can mean autistic adults – and sometimes children – get attacked for not being 'autistic enough'. There is a lot of division as the culture shifts from parent/carers dominating the narrative to autistic people having a powerful collective voice (Sanchez 2018). Even without these wider political/scientific considerations, there are other reasons why parent carer groups aren't the best environment for autistic people too – parents have to vent, complain and ask questions, but this can be hurtful to autistic people regardless of intention. Also any training, resources and support are often not 'geared' towards autistic needs, in content, pace and many other factors.

The autistic experience of breast/chestfeeding

The vast majority of maternity service users are women, identify as women and use the term 'breastfeeding' to describe feeding their baby breastmilk from the breast. However, numbers of referrals to gender identity services have risen exponentially over the last ten years (Tavistock and Portman NHS Foundation Trust 2019). This is important because almost two-thirds of the referrals are people who were assigned female at birth. In view of this, maternity services are moving towards using more inclusive language so that transgender (trans) and non-binary (including agender, bigender and genderqueer) people can see themselves in the service they use, such as maternity services. Research demonstrates that the way people are described impacts how they feel, and how likely they may or may not be to access a service (Jennings, Goût & Whittaker 2022). Can you imagine using a service that does not value who you are as a person, where the language used to define you does not apply to you? For this reason, using terms such as 'birthing person' or 'parent' instead of 'woman' or 'mother', and referring to 'chestfeeding' human milk instead of 'breastfeeding' breastmilk can offer individualised, personalised and holistic respectful care at a time of vulnerability and change. For this reason, these terms will be used interchangeably throughout the following content about feeding.

Breastfeeding has been a significant part of motherhood since time began. This is evident from the plethora of breastfeeding art ranging from oil paintings created in the 1500s, large sculptures constructed in the 1600s, photographs from the Victorian era, right up to modern-day art too. Chestfeeding can be as much a part of the mother–baby journey as it has been throughout history as human milk is tailor-made for each individual baby's requirements for nutrition, immunity and lifelong health. However, whether a birthing person breast/chestfeeds or not is not as simple a choice as it would seem.

The barriers to chestfeeding success originate from a myriad of factors such as social, medical, psychological, physical, cultural, commercial, political, geographical, economic and societal, to name but a few! The point here is that feeding success appears dependent upon the choices people make;

however, those choices are highly influenced by factors outside an individual's control. One such factor is evident in the work of the International Baby Foods Action Network (IBFAN) who have worked since 1979 to ensure companies engaging in the misleading advertisement of infant formula are held to account. Infant formula has been in existence since 1867; however, when sales began to fall during the 1960s, third-world countries in Asia, Africa and South America were targeted by formula companies who promoted formula as being better for babies than breastmilk. Representatives dressed in nurses' uniforms gave parents free samples, doctors were paid to promote the milk, and for the mothers who used the formula, their breastmilk ceased. Many parents could not afford the formula and they did not have access to clean water or sterilising equipment, which led to many babies dying of malnutrition and diarrhoea (IBFAN 2020). This is simply one example of how feeding is determined by much more than the birthing person.

Feeding success for many is also largely dependent upon the support they receive in the early postnatal period, and this is especially important for autistic people. Grant *et al.* (2022) suggest that feeding knowledge and determination was high in the sample of autistic women they spoke to; however, positive breastfeeding experience was only reported by a minority. Analysis of the data collected identified that 'maternity and infant feeding services were built on a lack of understanding autistic needs and were often inaccessible at a time when autistic mothers already felt a loss of control and lack of social support' (Grant *et al.* 2022). Autistic people found that sensory challenges, pain and interoceptive differences were exacerbated by a lack of support, which made breastfeeding impossible for some. For those who used infant formula instead, only a minority found the ritual of preparing bottles a positive experience. When the feeding method of choice is not as expected, a magnitude of emotions and feelings such as loss, failure, guilt and shame can ensue, which is an extremely poor start to parenthood for those people. Grant *et al.* (2022) therefore suggest there is an urgent need to redesign maternity and infant feeding service provision and train staff to accommodate autistic needs.

Case studies
Hayley shares her own experience of breastfeeding:

> With my first pregnancy, I had a very difficult experience with breastfeeding. About halfway through my pregnancy, at one of my appointments I

mentioned to the consultant that I had been lactating colostrum intermittently – particularly when emotionally stimulated (e.g. deep empathy for a partner or a crying baby on TV). The consultant expressed alarm and what I perceived to be some level of disgust. Around 24 weeks gestation, I was told by a consultant registrar in the hospital that I should start collecting and freezing colostrum in a pre-emptive effort to bank this precious resource for my baby. This advice was given as I had been diagnosed with gestational diabetes (GD) – something that affected both my pregnancies but was controlled with diet, exercise activity and metformin tablets with large meals. I struggled immensely with this and didn't have enough information and equipment to store the tiny amounts of colostrum correctly. So, when baby was born, due to the GD, baby was fed with formula to monitor his blood sugar levels effectively as is protocol for the condition. When I asked for help with initiating breastfeeding, I had a rather rough encounter with a ward visit from the lactation nurse/midwife. She aggressively took my breast and demonstrated the correct motions for getting colostrum out – I think this was with the view that I would only be feeding the baby expressed milk from a bottle, despite telling staff that I wanted to breastfeed exclusively. When I got home after the C-section, I cried on the phone to my sister-in-law that I couldn't get the baby to latch correctly. As she was in her second year of training to be a midwife and is autistic herself, she was a fantastic help in teaching me the easiest ways to hold and latch baby on. The following day, I proudly told the midwife at the home post-op visit that I had struggled but was making progress on starting my breastfeeding journey while temporarily 'topping up' with formula feeds until my milk supply was sufficient. The midwife told me that what I was doing, in trying to establish breastfeeding a few days after birth, was 'selfish, cruel and not fair on the baby' as he 'had already had a teat from a bottle'. Those words stayed with me forever as breastfeeding was something I'd always imagined doing; the baby would root for a nipple furiously and I had been told trying to latch him on was 'cruel'. In the end, I went against medical advice and persisted. Baby and I taught each other and by six weeks old we had a lovely breastfeeding journey together until he was 18 months old when he self-weaned. I went to breastfeeding support groups in my local area but found the room a complete sensory overwhelm, despite the comforting, anchoring aspect of breastfeeding.

With my second baby, I was prepared with more knowledge and experience. I was also self-diagnosed and on the waiting list for an autism assessment. I was sure of myself and my abilities as a mother. Baby instantly latched on and we breastfed until he self-weaned at 2–2.5 years.

Feeding guidance for mothers in the UK recommends exclusive breast- or chestfeeding for the first six months followed by human milk in addition to solid food thereafter (UNICEF/NHS 2022). Some mothers, like Hayley, are successful in this, especially with second and subsequent children. Some autistic mothers will choose to feed their baby with formula (or artificial milk as referred to by midwives), especially those who think literally. This is because, for them, formula feeding means they can monitor and measure how much milk the baby is receiving, although they must be advised how to recognise when formula volumes must increase. This is not to say that there is no way to monitor or measure chestfeeding. Feeds are measured by the number of feeds over a 24-hour period, the amount of time taken to feed, and monitoring the signs of a well baby, which include waking for feeds, sleeping between feeds and weight gain. Feeding options can be explored with parents in pregnancy, and it is important for health professionals to consider the needs of autistic women when offering advice.

Eating and sharing food is typically viewed as a social activity or at least an accepted activity. However, when it comes to breastfeeding in public spaces, in the words of Amy Brown (2021) this may be viewed by some as 'breast is best, but we don't want to see that'. I think we have all heard stories about women who have been tutted at, glared at or asked to leave a public café despite breastfeeding being protected by law under the Equality Act 2010.

Boyer (2018) proposes that breastfeeding women are expected to act in ways which maintain public comfort or risk disapproval. Breastfeeding, for some, is not considered to belong in public spaces and this can be understood through the 'male gaze' and through two foundations of patriarchy – the first that care work or 'women's work' belongs in the home and the second that women's bodies are considered to function for the sexual pleasure of men, whereby the display of sexualised breasts is vulgar (Boyer 2018). Such attitudes can lead to an 'intangibility of atmosphere' where the discomfort of others is felt rather than seen, which can lead women and birthing people to feel that they don't belong and certainly should not feed in such spaces. Thankfully, not all people feel like this, and some women are pleasantly surprised by the positivity demonstrated towards them in public places and feel that their confidence in breastfeeding in public spaces grows alongside general chestfeeding confidence and feelings of success.

Some women do feel uncomfortable breastfeeding in public because of gender-based marginalisation and a fear of disapproval from strangers. Retailers feed into this school of thought and compound such issues by offering 'breastfeeding' clothes, capes, hoods, covers, cushions and blankets whose sole purpose is to offer discretion when chestfeeding. Lactation rooms and combined feeding and nappy changing rooms also compound this idea, which, actually, is an improvement on when I (Karen) used to use public toilets to feed my first and second baby. When I had my subsequent three children, I felt more confident in my ability to breastfeed and did so in public without a second thought. Because I experience sensory overload, I would not have been able to feed my baby if I felt I had to cover myself with a hood or have the stress of learning how to use and wear 'breastfeeding' clothes. Such overwhelm can cause anxiety for autistic people and and they may not consider chestfeeding as a result. I think the message needs to be clear for women: they do not need to cover themselves with such items in public if they don't want to. Breastfeeding is protected in law and thankfully not all parents feel uncomfortable; some find it empowering and freeing, as described by Hayley:

> I found it incredibly freeing – embracing my autistic identity and the fact I don't adhere to many social norms and expectations meant that breastfeeding in public came with ease. This was quite freeing. The release of oxytocin meant that breastfeeding was an instant cocoon of calm and relief from sensory overload – even in the busiest shopping centres.

This is such a powerful statement from Hayley as it demonstrates how the oxytocin produced for milk ejection (or let-down) can have a calming effect on the woman too. This is because oxytocin blocks cortisol, and so for many women, if they are supported and understood, chestfeeding can be enjoyable.

> I'd given birth via emergency C-section a couple of hours previously after days of labour. I was exhausted but comforted by the stillness and darkness of the hospital at night. Keen to start breastfeeding, I was nervously excited when my baby cried out for food for the first time. I was alone and on no pain relief after the operation, so I pressed the buzzer for help from staff. The staff member, intentionally or unintentionally, put the help

button out of reach behind the bed. Every time my baby cried, I couldn't physically reach him and now couldn't ask for help – I sat and sobbed as he screamed for food. He's eight years old now and has never slept away from me, I go cold with panic when a new situation requires him to be somewhere new or further away – the thought of not being able to 'get to him' all over again takes over and I'm back to that moment.

Hayley

Karen's experience of breastfeeding and supporting mothers to feed

Similar to Hayley's experience, I was excited to breastfeed my first baby but was unprepared for how it would feel to hold a baby and latch a baby on to the breast. Back in 1991, the support I received was from a midwife twisting my breast into my baby's mouth which was painful. I lasted three weeks before giving up, which I felt guilty about. When I had my second baby, I was supported by a breastfeeding supporter who visited me at home, which also made it easier for me to attend a breastfeeding support group as I had met the supporter in my home first. As a midwife, my experiences helped shape the support I give to women. I feel that because breastmilk is natural, women assume that the breastfeeding skill will come naturally and are disappointed when it is difficult. Like all new skills, these need to be learnt and if women have not breastfed before, simply holding a baby in a good position for breastfeeding can take time to learn and coordinate. I think that if birthing people understand this is a new skill which both mother and baby need to practise, they may be less likely to feel they have failed at breastfeeding if it is difficult to establish.

Babies who have been solely chestfed are held by their caregivers differently and have a different sucking mechanism compared to babies who are fed solely through a teat. If a baby has been fed by a bottle at birth for reasons such as the need to maintain blood sugar as Hayley mentioned, the mother may need support to adjust the way they hold the baby for feeding, and the baby may need support with latching correctly to the breast to feed. Babies can learn to feed differently between breast and bottles, plus women are able to recognise the difference a good latch can make when they know what signs to look for. Parents often are not informed that mixed feeding is achievable, albeit with difficulty at first, and so have the idea that feeding should only be through one method only, which is incorrect. If people wish to feed their baby through methods such as alternating between human milk and artificial milk, then their choice can be supported by providing them with the information to do this effectively, such as expressing milk to continue the supply and learning how to prepare milk and sterilise equipment safely.

Chestfeeding is recommended for all babies, but this may be difficult for some, especially those with a sensory processing difficulty, and so feeding expressed breastmilk may be a good alternative. Most of the hospitals in the UK follow the UNICEF Baby Friendly Initiative (2019), which sets out the standards for supporting good infant nutrition and the promotion of close relationships between parents and babies. The standards include education for those who discuss feeding choices with women and birthing people, with the idea that they all receive the same guidance regarding infant feeding. Of course, within this are the individual experiences of the professionals, and so some advice may still differ from professional to professional. For autistic people, this can be confusing, which may lead to them not knowing who to listen to. This may inevitably lead to difficulties with feeding, and so continuity of carer and consistency of breastfeeding support from a limited number of people is essential. Hayley's experience demonstrates how the words professionals use can stay with women, and I am always mindful of this when I support parents myself. Words can have a profound effect on people's self-esteem and confidence, which can ignite feelings of failure for the current breastfeeding journey and affect subsequent breastfeeding attempts. I have seen the power kindness, patience and understanding can have on families, and this should be at the heart of any feeding support.

When supporting autistic women with infant feeding, whether that be breast, chest or alternative methods, altering your method of information sharing may be essential. I know that if I am told information in a noisy environment, I may not retain the information. Hospital and clinic environments can be brightly lit and noisy. Some alternatives could include visual tools such as videos or pictures, a list of instructions to refer to, and physical demonstrations where the parents can practise the new skill and have it checked. Chestfeeding supporters need to be providing 'hands-off' feeding support, which means that feeding techniques are often discussed or demonstrated with a knitted breast. Some people may still struggle with this and may ask you to be hands on. Being aware that some autistic women may experience heightened pain with touch is essential, and touch must only be used if requested, with the reiteration that they must tell you if it is painful as this may not be obvious to them. Of course, asking the parents how they learn best is always a good start.

Anecdotally, the early postnatal period is a difficult time for women to learn new skills, especially in the hospital environment, which is busy and where parents may feel pressured by the urgency of the task needed and babies crying. At the time of writing, most antenatal education in the UK is still not held face to face due to the Covid-19 pandemic, and, of course, not everyone feels comfortable learning in group settings. Information provided on the internet is not always consistent or evidence-based. Breast- and chestfeeding videos on YouTube may only discuss particular issues and not be relevant at all. Individualised antenatal education, therefore, may be beneficial for autistic parents to practise skills such as holding a baby for feeding (which could be using dolls), changing nappies, making up feeds and putting a breast pump together, and may mean they are able to learn these skills before their baby arrives in a calmer environment such as their home. Of course, not all autistic parents will need this support, but it is good to have this in mind.

Emma describes her experience of breastfeeding:

> My experience of breastfeeding started badly and we never quite made it successfully. After giving birth, I was able to shower and change. Then a midwife I didn't know entered my room, where myself, my partner and our new baby were staying, and there was another midwife and an additional member of staff in the room. The midwife that entered said something along the lines of 'Right, let's get your milk supply going' or 'Let's check your milk' and proceeded to reach down, open my nightie, take out my breast and begin expressing by hand into a kidney bowl. Already feeling ravaged by birth, vulnerable and shell-shocked, I just looked on, mute and paralysed. It had never felt more that my body did not belong to me. It was not the positive first experience I would have wished for, and looking back I think it was an egregious overlook of the importance of consent, amongst other things.

CHAPTER 3

Coexisting Conditions

This chapter will include information on commonly occurring coexisting conditions such as mental health, autoimmune disorders, sleep and eating disorders/disordered eating and more, and their impact on pregnancy, birth and new parenthood will be discussed.

- Overview

- Neurodevelopmental conditions

- Learning/intellectual disabilities

- Mental health

- Sleep problems

- Other conditions

- Autistic people in caring roles

- Medication

Overview

Is autism more systemic than we have previously believed? Does it affect multiple systems in the brain and body, including the brain and sensory, immune and autonomic nervous systems?

In recent years, an increasing number of researchers and clinicians have focused their attention on abnormalities of the autonomic nervous system (ANS) within the autistic population. This system helps control automated processes such as breathing, cardiac output, digestion, temperature and perspiration.

Elevated sympathetic and lowered parasympathetic activity is frequently present in autistic people, whether or not they have more obvious outward symptoms. The two branches are sometimes referred to as:

- sympathetic: fight, flight or freeze

- parasympathetic: rest and digest.

This correlates with the experiences that autistic people relate of meltdown and/or shutdown, which can be related directly to the fight, flight or freeze response, a survival mechanism designed to help humans survive potential threats or danger. In the case of those experiencing chronic or acute anxiety, known to be prevalent in the autistic population, these responses may be triggered more often and by a wider range of precipitating factors. This may also happen due to other autistic characteristics such as hypersensitivity to sensory information, social difficulties, past/accumulated trauma or intolerance of uncertainty, which may lead to perception of dangers that the general population would not perceive in the same way. It is further reinforced by the difficulties widespread in the autistic community with eating, digestion and sleep.

While we need further research on just how systemic autism truly is, it is clear that it rarely comes alone, with coexisting conditions being the norm for the majority of autistic people. Indeed, nearly three-quarters of children diagnosed with autism also have another medical or psychiatric condition, a statistic that can continue into or even increase in adulthood, with one chronic condition increasing the likelihood of another, and another, like a snowball rolling downhill (Raising Children 2022). Autistic people are likely to have one or more co-occurring conditions, such as mental health conditions, autoimmune diseases, eating disorders, dysautonomia, sleep and eating disorders, epilepsy and other neurodiverse conditions such as ADHD and dyspraxia (Isaksen *et al.* 2012).

These coexisting conditions can take a tremendous toll on the lives of autistic people and their families, increasing existing difficulties in behaviour, socialisation, sensory sensitivities and many aspects of daily life.

Because coexisting conditions are so common, it's important to understand how they can complicate autistic life, from making diagnosis more difficult to intensifying characteristics and difficulties. When we accurately diagnose and treat coexisting conditions, we can sometimes achieve improvements in understanding, management and quality of life for autistic people and their loved ones.

The impact of these conditions during pregnancy, birth and the postnatal period should be considered, and coping strategies developed, but currently many autistic women are without tailored support.

Because coexisting conditions are both so common and so vital to the overall picture when supporting an autistic person, this chapter will provide information on some of the most commonly reported coexisting conditions autistic people experience, and briefly explore the impact of both medication usage and potential cessation during pregnancy.

Neurodevelopmental conditions
Overview/unique different wiring

The co-occurrence of other neurodiverse conditions can complicate some of the difficulties autistic women may face, such as ADHD adding to struggles with time management and emotional regulation, and dyspraxia compounding motor and emotional difficulties (Croen *et al.* 2015).

ADHD

ADHD is a lifelong neurodivergent condition characterised by excess energy and difficulty concentrating. ADHD also presents difficulties with executive function, emotional regulation and impulse control, which can compound any difficulties already experienced in these domains by autistic people.

Signs of ADHD usually present very early in life, before the age of six, although some adults may have been missed or misdiagnosed. We don't know exactly what causes ADHD, but experts think it might run in families or it could be to do with the way the chemicals in your brain work.

Autism and ADHD often coincide, and there is much overlap between the two conditions. An estimated 30–80% of autistic children also meet the criteria for ADHD and, conversely, 20–50% of children with ADHD for autism. Obviously, this means adults also often have both conditions.

Learning/intellectual disabilities

Mitra and colleagues (2015) found that there were increased complications in pregnancy and birth in women with intellectual disabilities, including prolonged hospitalisation after delivery, pre-eclampsia, preterm birth, caesarean delivery and foetal death (after 20 weeks).

Mental health

Pre-existing mental health conditions such as anxiety, depression and obsessive compulsive disorder (OCD) could be exacerbated by the stress of pregnancy and birth, and can be an indicator for birth trauma, PTSD-PC and PND (Mannion & Leader 2013; McGonigle 2014; Meier *et al.* 2015; Verrault *et al.* 2012).

> Approximately 70% of the autistic population has at least one, if not multiple, co-occurring mental health issues...numbers might be higher in adults, as social anxiety and depression often emerge during adolescence and are more common in adolescents with autism than in those with other types of disabilities. (Roux & Kerns 2016)

Anxiety and depression (state and trait)

Anxiety and depression can be either states or traits. State relates to stressful/worrying situations and circumstances, whereas trait is inherent to the person and may persist regardless of external triggers. Many autistic people may experience high levels of both forms of anxiety and/or depression.

Self-injurious behaviours and suicidality

- 50% of the autistic population will engage in self-injurious behaviour at some point in their lives.

- Self-injurious behaviours are often related to anxiety, stress and frustration.

- Autistic adults are more than nine times more likely to consider suicide than the general population.

- This number has been reported as even higher in what is sometimes termed 'high-functioning' autism – as much as 16 times that of the general population.

- Children with autism are 28 times more likely to think about or attempt suicide.

- The mortality rate of the autistic population is twice that of the non-autistic population.

- Self-harm and suicidality have been linked to the impact of 'masking' in recent research (Camio *et al.* 2011 in Botha & Frost 2020).

(Steenfeldt-Kristensen, Jones & Richards 2020)

PTSD/complex PTSD

Autistic people seem to be more likely to experience/accumulate trauma. This is potentially because:

- they are often vulnerable

- they find things traumatic which others may not.

Remember that it is the perception of danger/threat that is key in experiencing trauma, and potentially developing post-traumatic stress disorder (PTSD) or complex PTSD (CPTSD). For example, a hand dryer starting unexpectedly could be a traumatic event for a noise-sensitive autistic child – leading to them avoiding all public bathrooms in the future.

Dissociation and dissociative identity disorder (DID)

Autistic people may experience dissociative states when in shutdown or meltdown. This can also occur due to coexisting mental health conditions, stress or anxiety. It can also happen in response to the effects of alcohol, drugs and some medication, or withdrawal from these.

A specific condition which goes beyond dissociative episodes is dissociative identity disorder (DID). This disorder is when a person has two or more identities/selves living within themselves. They may identify as living as a system or unit.

This fracturing of self often occurs as a result of trauma, as a coping/protective mechanism. As a person with this disorder described it, 'I felt like my body didn't belong to me, it was like I was an outsider watching my own story unfold' (Mind 2023).

Obsessive compulsive disorder (OCD)

- OCD is a condition that means a person becomes fixated on repetitive and stereotyped behaviours.

- Research suggests that OCD is more common among teens and adults with autism than it is in the general population.

- However, it can be difficult to distinguish OCD symptoms from the repetitive behaviours and intense interests that are characteristic of autism.

- Between 8% and 24% of autistic people have OCD, compared to just 1.2% of the total UK population.

(Autism West Midlands 2020; Yuhas 2019)

Bipolar disorder (BPD)

People with bipolar disorder tend to alternate between a frenzied state known as mania and episodes of depression.

Some autistic people are misdiagnosed with bipolar due to the overlap of how characteristics can present, although it is possible for the conditions to coexist.

It is important to distinguish the symptoms of true bipolar disorder from those of autism by looking at when the symptoms appeared and how long they lasted. For example, an autistic child may be consistently high-energy and overly social through childhood. As such, her tendency to talk to strangers and appear hyper/enthusiastic is likely related to her autism and not a symptom of a manic mood swing. As described by one person with bipolar disorder:

> The hardest thing about living with autism and bipolar is that most people remember me by my meltdowns rather than what I'm good at. It upsets me because I'm more than a person with problems and I wish people will just see that. (Mind 2015)

Schizophrenia

Autism and schizophrenia both involve challenges with processing language and understanding other people's thoughts and feelings.

Clear differences include schizophrenia's psychosis, which often involves hallucinations. In addition, autism's core characteristics typically emerge at ages 1–3 years (although recognition and diagnosis can happen much later); schizophrenia emerges in early adulthood.

Autism and schizophrenia co-occur significantly more often than would be expected by chance, with a study collating results from 2 million people finding it to be 3.6 times as common in autistic people (Chisholm *et al.* 2015). Autism likewise occurs more often in people with schizophrenia than in the general population.

Researchers have long suspected that autism and schizophrenia are related. The two conditions have overlapping traits, including sensory-processing problems and social difficulties, and they share gene expression patterns in brain tissue.

Some people have been misdiagnosed, or have been correctly diagnosed with one mental health condition with no further investigation into other potential conditions such as autism, perhaps due to the overlap and complexity in these conditions, and perhaps due to autistic characteristics such as echolalia, scripting, masking or the adoption of differing accents – most commonly American accents – being misinterpreted as signs of personality or dissociative disorders or schizophrenia. Jennifer Foss-Feig, assistant professor of psychiatry at the Icahn School of Medicine at Mount Sinai in New York, has said, 'Regardless of the way we look at it – schizophrenia in autism or autism in schizophrenia – the overlap between the two disorders is higher than we'd expect' (Gholipour 2018).

Personality disorders

There are reports of autistic women especially being misdiagnosed with borderline personality disorder (BPD), due to the similarity in characteristics in some cases.

- 68% of autistic people met DSM-IV criteria for at least one personality disorder.

- Six out of 41 BPD patients fulfilled criteria for autism.

(Dudas et al. *2017)*

Addiction

There are several potential risk factors for addiction in the autistic population, including:

- self-medication

- impulse control difficulties

- emotional dysregulation

- difficulty anticipating consequences of actions

- mimicry

- risky behaviour

- mental health conditions

- ADHD.

Addiction can take many forms, including:

- alcohol

- drugs

- food

- gaming.

More research is being done on autism and addiction, but we need to be aware of the risks and how to mitigate them.

Disordered eating and eating disorders

Eating disorders such as anorexia and avoidant/restrictive food intake disorder (ARFID) are common in autistic women and could impact massively during the perinatal period on both mother and baby, mother's mental and emotional wellbeing, and success/duration of breastfeeding (Kimmel *et al.* 2015; Mandy & Tchanturia 2015).

Studies have reported eating and feeding problems to be present in as many as seven out of ten autistic people, with autistic traits also being common in those with eating disorders – between 4.7 and 22.9%. Anorexia has been shown to be present in nearly a quarter of autistic females across several studies on the topic (NAS 2021b). Conversely, one London clinic found that one in four of those females in treatment for anorexia met the cutoff for autism when screened, suggesting there is a substantial link between the two conditions, and that autism 'might be a particular risk factor for developing a restrictive eating disorder' (Arnold 2016).

Autistic people are also more likely to experience food intolerances, sensitivities and allergies, including irritable bowel syndrome. Even without a specific diagnosis, the ties between autism and gastrointestinal issues are well-documented, with many autistic people suffering with diarrhoea, constipation and even lazy bowel and faecal impaction, particularly where there is a coexisting learning disability (Grant *et al.* 2022; Madra, Ringel & Margolis 2020).

What is also clear is that the underlying drivers for disordered eating or specific eating disorders can potentially be attributable to: sensory sensitivities, prior sensory trauma around food, need for control, associative memory links, rigidity of thought, anxiety, central autonomic nervous system differences (i.e. elevated fight–flight–freeze and lowered rest-and-digest responses), emotion dampening (i.e. lack of adequate nutrition can dampen our ability to feel emotions and anxiety), to stave off puberty due to a mismatch in our social, emotional and physical development or due to gender identity differences and intense interests around food, nutrition, categorising and the numbers relating to calories, fat, carbohydrates, sugars and so on. Autistic people often experience a lack of control in their daily lives, being bombarded by sensory information externally, and so food intake can be the one thing they feel able to control (NAS 2021b).

It is vital not to teach compliance around food as this may also teach a lack of bodily autonomy in other situations, as well as potentially making the relationship with food and eating hostile, compounding existing restrictive eating. Restricted eating or overeating can also be a form of self-injurious behaviour where there are coexisting mental health conditions.

Recovery from eating disorders may look different for autistic people, and it is important to be aware of the need for differentiated approaches because of this, particularly as pregnancy could be a difficult time for those experiencing restrictive food disorders. It is worth professionals visiting the PEACE pathway website for more information on this topic (PEACE 2020).

Emetophobia may be a particular difficulty during pregnancy too – if morning sickness is prevalent, it could pose additional problems due to this phobia.

Sleep problems

Sleep is one of the four main biological drives, along with eating, drinking and reproducing. Despite this, sleep remains much of a mystery, with sleep scientists still searching for definitive answers as to why we sleep. What is clear, however, is that sleep is vital for humans to remain healthy and functional, and that sleep deprivation can have significant negative consequences.

Sleep, however, is of key concern to many autistic people and their families, with studies suggesting up to 80% of autistic adults experience some form of sleep disturbance (Summer & Adavadkar 2023).

Why is sleep affected in autistic people?

- Central/autonomic nervous system abnormalities (see the overview for this chapter).

- Sensory issues – sensitivity to light, sounds, smells and touch can play a part in disrupting quality and duration of sleep.

- Different circadian rhythms and melatonin levels:

  - Research shows that autistic people have different circadian rhythms and differences in melatonin production (Tordjman *et al.* 2015)

  - It seems that there is a possible genetic link between gene mutations linked to circadian rhythms, sleep difficulties and autism.

  - In fact, autistic people are twice as likely to carry alterations in genes that regulate the sleep–wake cycle.

  - This can explain why as, one researcher suggests, in the case of autistic children, although they may tend to not be very social during the day, once it's time to go to bed 'all of a sudden, they're more social; they're happier, they want to play with a toy they never want to play with' (Chen 2015).

  - Researchers identified as many as 33 'missense' gene mutations, eight of which appeared to be damaging to the sleep process (Nuwer 2015).

  - These differences in sleep patterns can also exist in those with ADHD.

  - Unfortunately, there is societal stigma around being a 'night owl' as opposed to the celebrated 'early bird', although this is often predetermined and outside an individual's control.

- Overactive/hyperactive brain and body, anxiety, need for control – or perhaps most relevant in terms of sleep, a difficulty relinquishing control. Sleep could be viewed as the ultimate loss of control:

  - Anxiety is a factor that causes sleep difficulties in many people. Anxiety is so common in autistic people, with up to 84% experiencing anxiety (McGonigle *et al.* 2014), that this is often a big part of sleep problems.

  - A busy brain related to autism, ADHD and/or anxiety can make this even more difficult – with racing looping thoughts making it really hard to wind down and settle to sleep.

- A busy brain and anxiety throughout the day can also contribute to restless sleep and vivid dreams as we attempt to process this backlog as we sleep.

- In autistic people, particularly those with demand-avoidant profiles, sleep is not only a demand but also the ultimate loss of control.

- When we are hypervigilant, sleep is the last thing on our mind – and the central nervous system differences we see in autistic people can mean it is hard for them to feel safe enough to sleep.

- This makes sense when we see altered sleep patterns where autistic people sleep during the day when trusted loved ones are awake – it could potentially be an unconscious form of threat reduction, much as humans would sleep in shifts when vulnerable to predators and other dangers to conserve the safety of the family unit or community.

• Other coexisting conditions including gastrointestinal issues, mental health and chronic pain.

• Lifestyle factors such as diet and exercise.

• Social cues as well as knowing how and when to sleep, and how long for.

• Negative associations with sleep (e.g. nightmares).

As a result, disordered sleep and even sleep disorders are common in autistic people, including:

• REM sleep percentage reduction

• insomnia

• bruxism

• nocturnal enuresis

• nightmares

• night terrors.

The potential effects of sleep difficulties on autistic people include:

• more repetitive behaviours

- more social and communication difficulties

- daytime fatigue

- irritability

- more hyperactive and easily distracted

- impact on emotions and mood

- negative impact for family unit as whole

- difficulties with learning and memory – factors such as insomnia, differing circadian rhythms and a reduction in melatonin result in overall sleep deprivation. This impacts on executive function not just in terms of using existing skills but also in the ability to embed new ones. Sleep plays a very important role in memory consolidation (i.e. transferring our short-term memories from that day's USB drive into the correct locations in our main hard drive – where sleep is disrupted, this process is also disrupted, meaning memory formation and retention can be affected.

When you consider that these underlying difficulties common in autistic people may be exacerbated by pregnancy, potentially causing additional fatigue, this is another factor that may impact overall wellbeing (Devnani & Hegde 2015).

It is clear that sleep difficulties both during pregnancy and whilst adjusting to life with a newborn could be a real cause for concern in autistic people.

Other conditions

There are several other conditions that seem to be more commonly reported by autistic people and may impact autistic health, pregnancy and birth, including:

- dysautonomia/postural tachycardia syndrome (PoTS)

- premenstrual dysphoric disorder (PMDD), endometriosis and polycystic ovary syndrome (PCOS), which can impact fertility, thus not only increasing difficulties with menstruation, mood and pain levels but also complicating the experience of pregnancy/becoming pregnant

- allergies.

Autistic people have increased likelihood of other conditions, such as epilepsy, autoimmune and gastrointestinal disorders, diabetes, heart disease and recurrent infections (Croen *et al.* 2015; Davignon *et al.* 2018; Thomas *et al.* 2017), while research suggests that general multimorbidity is becoming increasingly common, numbers in England rising from 1.9 million in 2008 to 2.9 million by 2018 (Department of Health 2012). This can lead to a complex patient profile, potentially indicative of lack of or inappropriate preventative care, with implications for future care and pain management.

Epilepsy

Epilepsy is a condition that affects the brain. When someone has epilepsy, they can have seizures. These are caused by a sudden burst of brain activity which temporarily stops the brain working properly. There are lots of different types of epilepsy and many possible causes.

Increased prevalence of epilepsy, which affects only 1–2% of the general population, has been reported in autistic people, ranging from 4% to 38% (Thomas *et al.* 2017). Autistic people who also have a learning disability are at particularly high risk and their epilepsy can be difficult to manage.

Autistic people often are not diagnosed with epilepsy until later in life than the general population, with epilepsy frequently not being identified until the teenage years or even later. People on the autism spectrum may have a different pattern of seizures in the brain. It may be harder to treat their epilepsy with drugs that work in the general population.

Epilepsy is now the leading cause of death in autistic people with a co-occurring learning disability (Autistica 2016), so it's vital to think carefully about how we keep people safe and well, being vigilant for red flags that may include unexplained staring spells, involuntary movements, unexplained confusion and severe headaches, whilst also considering less specific signs such as sleepiness or unexplained changes in abilities or emotions.

Gastrointestinal problems

Many autistic people report gastrointestinal difficulties which can include conditions such as:

- irritable bowel syndrome (IBS)

- constipation

- lazy bowel

- faecal impaction

- Crohn's disease

- inflammatory bowel disease (IBD)

- food intolerances.

Immune system disorders/chronic pain

Many autistic people and, in some cases, mothers of autistic children report experiencing one or more conditions that affect the immune/pain systems or cause chronic pain such as fibromyalgia, CFS/ME and lupus, all of which may complicate pregnancy, birth and parenthood, with a potential for a deterioration in these fluctuating conditions that could cause heightened pain, reduced energy levels and so on.

> I knew I would never cope with a second child. In many ways, it broke my heart and took a long time to accept, but my health conditions meant it was too risky to strain my family unit both with another pregnancy and birth, and with the additional taxation on energy levels a second child would inevitably introduce. I love my small family and am incredibly grateful to have experienced pregnancy, birth and to have our child, but I still feel no small amount of guilt for not feeling able to provide my much-loved child with a sibling, even if I know in my heart of hearts it is for the best.
>
> *Emma*

Ehlers–Danlos syndrome

Ehlers–Danlos syndrome (EDS) is a group of hereditary connective tissue disorders (HCTD). These affect the connective tissues (ligaments, tendons, skin, bone, blood, fatty tissue) which act like the glue that holds the body together. There are 13 types of EDS – 12 considered rare. The most common type is hypermobile EDS (HEDS).

Research is beginning to show strong links between autism and EDS, with studies finding that people with EDS are more likely to be autistic (Casanova *et al.* 2020). Also, autistic people are known to commonly experience joint hypermobility in general, a major feature of EDS.

Recent research found mothers with EDS or hypermobility spectrum disorders (HSD) are just as likely to have an autistic child as an autistic mother (Casanova *et al.* 2020). This suggests maternal EDS has a strong link with autism. EDS/HSD mothers with autistic children had more immune problems than EDS/HSD mothers without children on the spectrum. This may indicate that the mother's immune system has an important role.

Conditions such as EDS or hypermobility can also cause complications during pregnancy and birth in multiple ways, including slow wound healing, increased risk of dislocations/hyperextending joints and haemorrhage (Karthikeyan & Venkat-Raman 2018). This is covered in more detail in Chapter 4.

Autistic people in caring roles

Autistic people may also have a caring role. This likelihood may even be increased when we consider the genetic links in autism and other coexisting conditions, thus increasing the likelihood of children or other family members who are autistic or have other complex health needs.

Being a carer can also impact health and stress levels. Caring can also be physically demanding – for example, many carers have disturbed sleep as a result of caring, others have to help move or lift the person they are caring for.

The 2019 GP Patient Survey highlights the impact of caring on carers' health in England – whilst 51% of non-carers had a long-standing health condition, this rose to 63% of all carers, and 71% of carers caring for 50 or more hours a week (NHS England 2019a).

As well as the impact of a caring role on carer health, there seem to be some links to other conditions in family members – particularly mothers. There are many anecdotal reports of mothers of autistic children having autoimmune and related conditions, such as CFS/ME and fibromyalgia (Centers for Disease Control and Prevention 2018; Andersson 2021). EDS mothers also seem to have a higher incidence of having autistic children, as do mothers with gestational diabetes. Family history of mental health or other neurodivergent conditions is always considered in diagnosing someone with autism.

More investigation/research is needed, but there could be genetic links between certain conditions such as EDS and autism – or, potentially, the mothers with these conditions may have undiagnosed autism. It remains to be seen if either or both of these factors are true and more research into the complexities of health in autistic people and their biological relatives is needed.

Medication

During pregnancy, removal of existing medications may be indicated (Du Toit *et al.* 2015), such as SSRIs which often treat commonly co-occurring depression/anxiety (NICE 2009, 2011). Careful consideration – where possible, prior to pregnancy – should be given to any potential negative impact on the woman's mental, emotional and physical wellbeing due to withdrawal of such medications. Women may feel worry and stigma around the use of medications in pregnancy, especially if they suffer from heightened anxiety, and much of the information that floods your screen if you search for 'autism and medication' online focuses on prevention of autism and the risks of autism relating to medication use, which can be scary, emotionally difficult, and even devastating for autistic women to wade through.

CHAPTER 4

Pain and Sensory Differences

The interaction between sensory systems and pain in the autistic brain will be comprehensively discussed, as well as co-occurring conditions that may make this a significant disadvantage for the autistic birth experience. These may include alexithymia, chronic pain, Ehlers–Danlos syndrome and epilepsy. Recommendations will include newly devised pain scale approaches and descriptions of behaviours that may signal interoceptive pain or sensory overwhelm.

- Sensory differences
- Other sensory considerations
- Medication/anaesthesia/analgesia and differing sensor responses
- Hypermobility

Sensory differences

Autistic people have notable sensory differences, with multiple sensory systems often affected (Robertson & Baron-Cohen 2017). As discussed previously, autistic people may have a difference in processing sensory input from the environment. Research into lifelong struggles with pain have found a link between childhood hypersensitivity (particularly tactile) and chronic pain experienced from a younger age (Clarke 2015). This has the potential to be further compounded by the previously described difficulty with verbal communication that may present in immediate situations with sensory or pain stimulus present. This has the potential to have wider impact – for example, difficulty with communicating pain or other symptoms of chronic conditions – as well as a higher likelihood of having a distrust of medical care professionals.

Hadjikhani *et al.* (2014) found that autistic people showed similar levels of pain sharing and empathy activation to those of their neurotypical counterparts. However, a higher level of cognitive reappraisal was reported in autistic participants, suggesting that miscommunication of pain and empathy may be more likely to be caused by the autistic individual re-routing their thought process and reaction to others in pain. This is particularly pertinent to fathers, birth partners and others in the immediate support network, principally because they are more likely to be autistic themselves, whether formally diagnosed or displaying characteristics of the broad autistic phenotype (Richards *et al.* 2022). This may suggest that Milton's (2012) Double Empathy Problem is key to observing and interpreting autistic pain behaviours, as well as physiological evidence that masking is an inherent, neurological response hardwired into autistic people even in precarious/painful situations.

In mainstream practice, gauging the pain behaviour of patients may often require a pain scale tool to help the clinician and patient communicate. While there are many examples, and modifications are frequently being researched, most of these tools will fall into one of three categories – numerical rating scales, visual analogue scales and categorical scales.

Riquelme *et al.* (2016) found autistic participants to have an increased pain sensitivity particularly in regard to touch-sensitive areas – that is, c-tactile afferent innervated areas (hands, arms, head). This may result in an avoidance of touch and related behaviours.

Messmer (2008) states that 'caregivers may discount or deny signals of distress in [autistic] children who cannot clearly express their pain'.

Sensitivity to touch is a key concern in pregnancy and childbirth, due to atypical sensations throughout the body and the likelihood of regular physical examinations (Riquelme *et al.* 2016). Sensitivities to sight, sound and smell in a clinical environment may prove equally challenging, contributing to complete sensory overload in some cases (Hahn 2012; Nicholas *et al.* 2016).

Of key importance in childbirth, the experience of pain may be significantly altered in autistic people (APA 2013). There is some research on this topic that suggests potential underlying genetic differences, and altered pain responses, coping mechanisms and pain evaluation (Sener *et al.* 2017), although these have often been limited in scope or with conflicting results, and therefore further studies are necessary (Failla *et al.* 2017; Hadjikhani *et al.* 2014; Thaler *et al.* 2017). Individuals may experience hyper- or hypo-reactivity to pain, or a combination of both, with one study showing an abnormal response to pain in 25–40% of autistic people (Moore 2014). There is also a suggestion that this altered pain sensation and reaction may account for high levels of self-injurious behaviour in autistic people (Duerden *et al.* 2013; Minshawi *et al.* 2014; Summers *et al.* 2017).

Interoceptive awareness may be a key area for further study, with altered interoception suggested in autistic people, those with heightened anxiety and survivors of sexual trauma (Olthuis & Asmundson 2019; Price, Kantrowitz-Gordon & Calhoun 2019). Interoception is also said to play a role in caregiving during early parenthood (Abraham *et al.* 2019).

Responses from Morgan (2019) mirrored anecdotal reports from the autistic community, with 42.56% of autistic women agreeing they felt interoceptive bodily changes during pregnancy sooner than neurotypical peers or textbook information.

Expression/communication of pain may also be notably different. Alexithymia is an inability to identify and describe emotions in oneself and others and appears common in autistic people (Costa *et al.* 2017). Autistic people sometimes present a blunt or flat affect, rather than the usual facial and other expected expressions of pain (Faso, Sasson & Pinkham 2015).

Craig (2015) describes the socio-communicative model of pain (e.g. the communication of pain begins with the patient's experience of pain). Namely:

> 1) this experience influences the encoding of pain expressions, 2) these pain experiences are broadcast to observers, who then can decode the child's pain, 3) and potentially take action to alleviate the child's pain.

Arguably, a number of autistic people have the potential to be inherently excluded from a timely and sufficient response to their pain perception and communication. In this case, one could argue that evidence outlines an atypical processing at every stage of the socio-communicative pain process. For example:

- Alexithymia, masking and hypoactivity in limbic cortices caused by pain processing may not only have an effect on real-time pain communication as a contextless event but may indicate a deeper social suppression of pain reaction learned from childhood.

- Pain experiences are processed and communicated differently, if at all, resulting in an unreliable stimulus for caregivers and medical professionals.

- If the processing and communication is atypical, absent or asynchronous, the ability of medical staff to provide timely and sufficient analgesia is arguably dramatically reduced.

Consequently, professionals may not recognise distress or pain in autistic women during labour due to this atypical presentation (Allely 2013). It is imperative to realise that traditional pain measurement approaches (i.e. self-report and facial pain scales) may not be appropriate for autistic people. Studies also diverge in findings about expressivity of emotion – that it may be typical, exaggerated or fluctuate throughout the lifespan (Rattaz *et al.* 2013), though whether expressivity may have been learned or is just due to variance in the autistic population is unclear. Pain is important during birth in understanding progress and indicating complications, and not only impacts the mother but can affect the infant too (Labor & Maguire 2008; Maxwell, Watts Betser & David 2007). Healthcare professionals should remain mindful of varying degrees of expressivity and employ person-centred approaches. Women who feel their pain is understood and who feel empowered in their pain management choices report higher satisfaction and less distress (McCauley *et al.* 2018; Whitburn *et al.* 2019).

Other sensory considerations

Interoception gathers messages from throughout the body (i.e. organs, muscles, skin, bones, etc.) and sends them to the brain. The brain processes these messages and enables us to feel and identify sensations such as hunger, itchiness, pain, body temperature, nausea, need to urinate, etc. Additionally, interoception allows us to differentiate bodily sensations/needs from our emotions.

There are also specific conditions related to sensory differences which seem to be more prevalent in the autistic population, which will be described below.

Allodynia is described as a person feeling pain from something that shouldn't be painful at all, such as a very light touch. For a person not experiencing allodynia, undergoing a functional magnetic resonance imaging, and being pricked with a needle, a small spark would 'set off' in the brain. For a person experiencing allodynia, the same needle prick could result in a full fledged 'firework display' (He & Kim 2022).

Alexithymia can often include difficulties in identifying, describing and processing one's own feelings, or the feelings of others, and difficulty distinguishing between feelings and bodily sensations.

Synaesthesia is generally represented as when two or more of the five senses that are normally experienced separately are involuntarily and automatically joined together – for example, being able to 'taste' names, ticker-tape synaesthesia (where written words appear in the mind when listening, speaking or thinking), emotions having smells and so on.

Hyperacusis is the name for intolerance of everyday sounds that causes significant distress and affects a person's day-to-day activities. This is a generalised hypersensitivity and linked to the more well-known misophonia, which is a specific aversion to the sounds of other people breathing, chewing or swallowing, particularly in relation to food.

Medication/anaesthesia/analgesia and differing sensory responses

Pain processing and communication differences render this subject a matter of urgency. Research suggests that the autistic individual processes pain differently, skin and touch having hypersensitivity whether to touch from another person or to fabric (Griffin OT 2018), yet they have an overall higher tolerance of true interoceptive pain. The neurological response to pain stimulus also serves to intensify the already evidenced hypoactivity in the motor and limbic cortices, resulting in 'shutdown' or the inability to communicate (both verbally or physically).

In birth specifically, pain reporting during pregnancy and labour is key to safety, autonomy and overall wellness. Missed pain reporting potentially leads to negative consequences on morbidity and mortality (Flynn, Smith & Chou 2011).

There is some scant evidence that autistic people may have differing responses to medications, with peer-reviewed and anecdotal evidence suggesting the possibility of both hyper- and hyposensitivity across the lifespan, although one of these was conducted upon autistic mice, which raises concerns about the finding's validity in relation to human subjects (Kilbaugh *et al.* 2010; Li *et al.* 2017).

There is a clear need for further research in this area. This is of particular concern in maternity care: if analgesia and/or sedation may affect autistic people differently, this could have obvious effects during birth due to need, in some cases, for pain management and/or sedation (Van der Gucht & Lewis 2015). If caesarean or other surgery is needed, the effectiveness of anaesthesia is of utmost importance (Mankowitz *et al.* 2016). Common co-existing conditions may also have a significant impact on pain management and medication sensitivity, such as epilepsy, ADHD and other systemic conditions (Robbins & Phenicie 2011; Willner *et al.* 2014).

Hypermobility

A study found that autistic people were more likely to have subclinical symptoms (e.g. pain) as well as an official diagnosis of hypermobility (Casanova *et al.* 2018).

Casanova *et al.* (2020) found that 'individuals with average or above average cognitive ability tend to harbour a higher polygenic load of small effect variants which are often inherited and may also be linked with the BAP [broader autism phenotype] in parents and siblings'. Therefore, it is likely that more of the family and support network have presence of hypermobility joint syndrome (HJS) symptoms and may need diagnosis, signposting and support themselves.

A diagnosis of hypermobility is currently dependent on the affected person being observed to have joint hypermobility with a Beighton Scale 9 score and evidence against the efficacy of Beighton in HJS population (Bravo & Wolff 2006). With regard to complications from loose cartilage and deficiencies in collagen production, this has potential to impact autistic mothers with co-occurring EDS/HJS during pregnancy and birth. For example, symphysis pubis dysfunction (SPD), characterised by pain in the pelvic girdle and experienced by 20% of all pregnant women (Royal College of Obstetricians and Gynaecologists 2015), could potentially be worsened by pre-existing weaknesses in collagen, and may be compounded by pregnancy-related hormonal changes. For example, the hormone relaxin, which peaks in the first trimester and before delivery with the aim of loosening joints for accommodating a growing baby, may be more likely to affect autistic women with EDS/HJS (Kanakaris, Roberts & Giannoudis 2011). However, a causal relationship across all three variables has yet to be established.

Both the clinical and individual-level importance of chronic pain and hypermobile joint syndrome have arguably had little consideration as a systemic problem worthy of antenatal planning and consideration.

> Over the subsequent three decades its benign nature (at least as far as life expectancy is concerned) became apparent as the multi-systemic nature of the condition became better appreciated. However, it is only within the last ten years that its preeminent position as one of the major causes of chronic pain has become apparent... Yet even today, its importance to rheumatology

still eludes many of our clinical colleagues…and the resultant suffering goes largely unchallenged in both children and adults. (Hakim & Grahame 2003)

This predisposition to chronic pain may mean that autistic women experience

> a complex relationship that occurs with disturbances of higher central pain processing and psychosocial function…it is also clear that many individuals with HJS suffer from a number of other apparently non-specific symptoms such as fainting, palpitations, and gastrointestinal disturbance which may lead to secondary anxiety. (Smith 2017)

During pregnancy, specifically the abdominal and pelvic structures may be affected by HJS, 'resulting in an intrinsic weakness or poor tensile strength in supporting structures' (Smith 2017). This has potential to affect the rate of progression during labour as well as likelihood to experience SPD and delayed or difficult recovery postpartum. Research suggests those with HJS have pelvic floor weakness, leading to incidence of uterine prolapse as high as 40–60% (Norton & Baker 1995) . There are also increased rates of 'urinary incontinence, dyspareunia, hysterectomy and pelvic floor prolapse' in this population compared to unaffected women in the same age range (Smith 2017).

HJS also presents a 'risk of divarication of the rectus abdominis muscles as well as potential for trauma to the vaginal vault and surrounding soft tissues during labour, aggravated by poor wound healing' and 'labour tends to be more rapid' but whether this increases likelihood of trauma has yet to be confirmed with research (Smith 2017).

During pregnancy, there is a link between EDS/HJS and a 'premature rupture of the foetal membranes and possible antepartum haemorrhage' (Smith 2017).

Some hormonal contraceptives (whether used for contraception or other medical indications, such as acne or PMDD) increase hypermobility of joints (HMSA 2014; Bird & McIver 2014, cited in Smith 2017). There is seemingly a broad spectrum of effects of the interaction between joint hypermobility and pregnancy. Some people have reported few problems, while others have reported feeling pregnancy-related health problems much earlier or more intensely than their non-hypermobile peers (Smith 2017).

According to Sundelin *et al.* (cited in Smith 2017), 'EDS/HSD was not associated with any increased risk of preterm birth, the need for caesarean section, stillbirth, complications in the infant at delivery (a low Apgar score) or the infant being small or large for gestational age'. Hugon-Rodin (2016) (cited in Smith 2017) found higher risk of spontaneous abortion in the HJS population (28%) compared to the typical population (10–20%).

Some HJS women may experience worsening levels of hip and back pain during pregnancy; some may feel better than they did before. This is due to the individual response to hormones in pregnancy (e.g. oestrogen, relaxin). For example, in some people the hormones may worsen hip laxity and increase pain, whereas for others it may induce positive mood changes and decreased pain receptor sensitivity (Smith 2017).

While there are no official guidelines that midwives and doctors have to follow for patients presenting with HJS during pregnancy, they can still adapt care or refer to an obstetrician. According to the Ehlers-Danlos National Foundation:

> In connection with natural delivery, women with EDS have experienced incontinence, weak pelvic floor, prolapse of the uterus, sprained joints of the pelvis, separation of the symphysis pubis (the joint between the two pubic bones in the frontal lower part of the pelvis) and rupture of the rectal musculature. (Ehlers-Danlos National Foundation 2015, cited in Smith 2017)

Despite research showing a heterogenous, individualised physical response to HJS effects in pregnancy, the authors argue that more research is needed in this area, particularly regarding long-term complications that may severely impact health and wellbeing and the likelihood of becoming pregnant again in the future.

With regard to delivery, while research shows HJS women are no more likely to need a C-section, HJS may add additional risks to vaginal birth. Research has suggested a higher risk of unusually rapid delivery (Castori 2012; Charvet *et al.* 1991; Linf & Wallenburg 2002; Sorokin *et al.* 1994, all cited in Smith 2017).

Hypermobile joint syndrome, more likely to occur in autistic birthing people, is arguably of utmost importance when planning to care for autistic people in pregnancy birth. This has both short-term and long-term implications, for example potential escalation of contractions and subluxation of joints. Long term the chronic pain aspect of HJS may have implications to a birthing person's wellbeing and outlook on their pregnancy and motherhood.

Body temperature can be more dysregulated in pregnancy – there is potential for impact and sensitivity to this interoceptive unpredictability particularly for autistic people.

CHAPTER 5

Autistic Communication

Hayley's background is linguistics and she's very interested in the practical application of Milton's 'Double Empathy Problem' in this real-world setting. Practically speaking, this will take the form of a research-based foundation about autistic communication. This will then be built upon through the lens of double empathy, including approaches and tips to help bridge this gap between communication styles.

- Pragmatics and semantics

- Contemporary research at a glance

- Specific language difficulties/differences

Milton's Double Empathy Problem can be applied to the topic of communication, which, while a vast subject area, arguably has application in this real-world setting. For the purposes of this book, this will take the form of a research-based foundation through which we will explore autistic communication. This will then be built upon to include approaches and tips aimed at helping to bridge the gap between communication styles of neurotypical and autistic people.

At the very first point of recognising autistic traits, this may come in the form of early parental observations. Often parental reporting includes observations of limited eye contact, restrictive and repetitive behaviour (RRB)/stimming, 'extremes' of language including absence of speech, hyperlexia or phases of non-verbalism. Parents usually report to their health visitor or GP, and if the medical professional agrees with their observations/concerns at home, they will refer them for further assessment. Two of the most common characteristics to initiate the diagnostic process for parents of autistic children are a lack of joint attention gestures (protodeclarative gestures (PDG)) and a delay in social communication (Landa 2008).

Regarding the use of protodeclarative gestures, Samadi and McConkey (2015) found that when PDG-based behaviours were removed from the M-CHAT-R to create a culturally sensitive Iranian alternative, HIVA, it became a more sensitive screening tool. This raised the question of whether the 'autistic language culture' values PDG with the same importance as their neurotypical counterparts.

Throughout the lifespan, autistic people often present linguistic characteristics distinct from their typically developing peers – from lexicon acquisition to syntax differences (Tek *et al.* 2014).

Pragmatics and semantics

Co-occurring social and pragmatic 'disorders' are said to be more common in the autistic population. However, the Double Empathy Theory may add a shift in perspective from the deficit of the communication model in some instances. As an example, Grice's conversational maxims are shown in Table 5.1.

Table 5.1 The cooperative principles: maxims of conversations

Name of maxim	Description of maxim
Quantity	Say neither more nor less than discourse requires
Relevance	Be relevant
Manner	Be brief and orderly; avoid ambiguity and obscurity
Quality	Do not lie; do not make unsupported claims

Source: Grice 1991

Relational theory (Sperber & Wilson 1986) involves identifying (a) what the speaker intended to say, (b) what the speaker intended to imply, (c) the speaker's intended attitude to what was said and implied, and (d) the intended context.

Perspective: NT vs autistic response (based on a real example)

[silent bus stop]: 'This weather, eh?'

'My favourite thing is serial killers'

or

[acquaintance asks how you are in the supermarket]: 'Fine, thanks, yeah...'

'Why don't they turn the tannoy down? Ugh, I couldn't even find a parking space in my usual spot because this red Fiat was there, then the trolley wheel squeaked the whole way around. I don't want to take it back and get another one because there's too many people and I just want to get out as fast as I can...'

Crompton *et al.* (2020) found that interactions between autistic and non-autistic people are not as effective at transferring information as interactions between autistic peers.

We found a significantly steeper decline in detail retention in the mixed chains, while autistic chains did not significantly differ from neurotypical chains. Participant rapport ratings revealed significantly lower scores for mixed chains. These results challenge the diagnostic criterion that autistic people lack the skills to interact successfully. Rather, autistic people effectively share information with each other. Information transfer selectively degrades more quickly in autistic-with-neurotypical dyads, in parallel with a reduction in rapport.

Further work in this area has suggested 'relevance theory positions communication as contingent on shared – and, importantly, mutually recognised – "relevance". Given that autistic and non-autistic people may have sometimes markedly different embodied experiences of the world, we argue that what is most salient to each interlocutor may be mismatched' and 'Mutual understanding was unexpectedly high across all types of conversation pairings. In conversations involving two autistic participants, flow, rapport and intersubjective attunement were significantly increased' (Williams, Wharton & Jagoe 2021).

One could argue this strengthens the case for autism advocates, champions or autistic staff themselves to be involved in the care of autistic patients in order to better facilitate communication, consent and autonomy.

Contemporary research at a glance

Linked to Theory of Mind, protodeclarative gestures (PDG) are initially screened for (chronologically) during the M-CHAT-R tests undertaken by autistic children around 3–4 years of age, typically when parents first report atypical characteristics. This, in the UK, is most typically reported to a health visitor (HV), and the assessment is usually carried out by the HV with the parent and child present. Many of the behaviours are based on

PDG, which are, broadly, 'pointing' gestures. The underlying assumption here is that autistic people struggle to imagine the mindset and viewpoints of others and therefore there is an absence or atypicality of the behaviours that would normally demonstrate this. PDG has historically been reported as absent or delayed (Baron-Cohen 1989; Curcio 1978) or asynchronous and alternative (Özçalışkan, Adamson & Dimitrova 2016). Interestingly, Eigsti and De Marchena's research (2017) showed that PDG use in storytelling activities suggested an 'asynchronous and atypical' presentation. Again, there is an argument here that the Double Empathy Problem (Milton 2012) needs to be adopted for what is considered 'early symptoms' of autistic presentation, but also throughout the lifespan in terms of giving equal respect to an autistic communication style that develops differently to neurotypical counterparts.

Further investigation has indicated that autistic children use gestures for repetitive and self-regulatory purposes (Belger, Carpenter & Schipul 2014; Camaioni *et al.* 2003), which raises questions over the true motives of an autistic PDG and is of note particularly if observing a higher frequency of gestures in particular.

Boston University research suggests that as many as 30% of people with autism do not develop expressive language (Shield 2014); however, with the perspective of the Double Empathy Problem (DEP), one must consider how much research behind this fact holds true or whether they considered adjustments at all.

Research on emotion-word processing has suggested that emotionally charged language could amplify the hypoactivity of the motor and limbic cortices (Moseley *et al.* 2013) which, in the production of PDG, could play a role, for example, in deep special interests, interpersonal motivation and highly emotionally charged diagnostic assessments.

In terms of more immediate application of this phenomenon, it may be essential to a patient's wellbeing, autonomy and consent options to consider that there is an underlying linguistic/developmental difference causing the difficulty with productive speech rather than simply trying to alleviate perceived anxiety in the patient, etc.

Table 5.2 summarises examples of atypical communications and how they can be viewed from a DEP perspective.

Table 5.2 Atypical communications viewed from a DEP perspective

Example of atypical communication	DEP explanation and wider social model perspectives
Talking incessantly about one subject	Autistic people will offer or exchange facts (either about a topic they love or something in the environment) as a way of building rapport, similar to how neurotypicals respond to social small talk. In some situations, it's how autistic people will show empathy – by offering facts about their own experiences of similar situations. This may be seen as changing the topic or talking about themselves 'unnecessarily'.
Ability to communicate linked to anxiety	Research has suggested that the reduced or absent ability to communicate in autistic people is far more than a learned social anxiety response, but rather an inherent neurological mechanism. Hypoactivity in the limbic cortices is exacerbated as a stress response – that is, the speech and decision-making part of the brain in this scenario literally shuts down.
Using language confidently but lacking comprehension	This could be for a number of factors – sensory overwhelm, social anxiety, an interruption to script, processing delay, learning difficulties. This is particularly important to clinical settings – that is, they may script and communicate certain topics confidently but may in some circumstances be unable to give informed consent or participate in shared decision making, until comprehension is established.
Absence of any desire to communicate with others	This may initially be labelled non-verbalism. It may be due to the individual having a limited idiosyncratic lexion that doesn't apply to the clinical environments they find themselves in. It could also be a valid trauma response. It could also be processing delay, a lack of accommodations available (e.g. computer aid) or learning difference.
May not understand facial expressions and may misinterpret non-verbal communication	Common characteristics that you can find in any textbook about autism. However, it may be worthwhile framing this from another perspective (e.g. how are neurotypicals so sure they 100% know how other people are feeling inside?). It could be as a result of masking so long that they distrust the usefulness of facial expressions in others.
May not understand words or only seem to hear parts of sentences	Could be processing delay, language disorder, lack of accommodation for LD, distraction by sensory overwhelm.
Communication confined to the expression of needs only	In some cases, one could argue this is useful in clinical settings. However, for true person-centred care, we need to learn about the person's emotional responses, including fear, anxiety, confidence, unawareness, etc.

One-sided communication, difficulties with turn-taking, may interrupt	As mentioned above, this could be from showing empathy/ bond-building through sharing information or a script that has been practised beforehand. May be compounded by not reading facial or body language cues.
Literal interpretation, issues with verbal ambiguity	Autistic people can struggle with metaphor, idiom and other non-literal communication. Try speaking directly and without colloquialism wherever possible – this could arguably help all types of communication if adopted.
Use of 'scripts' or speaking as if learned by rote	In many cases, this is a robust coping mechanism that can be harnessed to great effect if adjustments are considered in place. This is a case of neurotypicals having to adjust their communication style somewhat. However, this is only if the scripts work in the situation and go to plan. Straying outside the script can be difficult, so chat in advance about what will happen at the next appointment (e.g. examinations, questions that will be asked).
Verbal stimming, repeating of stock phrases or sounds	Again, a valid coping mechanism to self-regulate from overwhelm. Familiarise yourself with them or wait for them to self-regulate enough to continue communicating.

Specific language difficulties/differences

- Often complete absence of speech, unreliable speech, repetitive speech and echolalia.

- Can confuse 'I', 'me', 'you' – this is a specific language disorder that may have implications for informed consent.

- Problems with pitch, tone, volume and intonation (this may be monotonous or seemingly inappropriate to the context of the utterance; there is also the propensity to have an unusual accent).

- Repetitive, stereotyped and inflexible use of words (generally a scripting thing or self-regulation but one must wonder how appropriate most neurotypical small talk is – it is in essence very repetitive and stereotyped and often rhetorical).

- Processing delay/problems (giving time, making questions known in advance if possible and allowing follow-up questions to be asked in another format – e.g. digital – could be helpful).

A number of these issues are illustrated by a book that is now (by some) associated with autism. *The Curious Incident of the Dog in the Night-Time*

(Haddon 2003) offers a first-person perspective of the experience of some of these social, semantic and pragmatic language differences. The author has stated that the book wasn't written specifically with autism in mind, but many individuals and families have found that it resonated with them deeply. Some of the language differences are illustrated by the following quote:

> people do a lot of talking without using any words…Siobhan…says that if you close your mouth and breathe out loudly through your nose it can mean that you are relaxed, or that you are bored, or that you are angry and it all depends on how much air comes out of your nose and how fast and what shape your mouth is when you do it and how you are sitting and what you said just before and hundreds of other things which are too complicated to work out in a few seconds… (Haddon 2003)

The poem 'Frozen' below was written by Hayley for the Swansea Autism Festival 2018 on the topic of a first-person account of reactive non-verbalism.

Frozen

Thrusting the tongue to resuscitate words
Like pulling spinach out of the sink
Eyes apologetically appealing
'Fill in the gaps'
Breath gone

Not aloof, passive or odd, but an understudy
Desperately proving ambivalence
Rehearsed in a second language
Lamenting my mother tongue
Mirror for survival

Irretrievable, unwanted decorum lost to the senses
Lips rescue the face, protesting synapses
Mind screaming expectations
Inescapable noisy light
Mouth curling passively

Forceful air seeks words for an acceptable communion
Sacrificing impulses to manifest mutuality
Mumbling, makeshift connections
Unmasking resisted
Play on

Eyes narrow to mimic a synthetic smile
Restless soul betrayed for now
Daily dance of gestures complete
Body slumps to a 'sorry'...
'So how is Mum doing?'

CHAPTER 6

Advice for Professionals

In this chapter, we will bring together all the topics discussed in earlier chapters and consider the impact this can have on professional practice, including standards of care such as the NMC code. Hayley will also present findings from her original research and Emma will present her proposed training plan for healthcare professionals.

- Your responsibilities and how autism impacts them

- Creation of a training package for midwives/healthcare professionals

- Practical advice and strategies

- Supporting autistic people with gender identity differences

- Wellbeing indicators and screening for postnatal depression

- Resources and tailored information

Your responsibilities and how autism impacts them
The Nursing and Midwifery Council (NMC) code
Prioritise people
You put the interests of people using or needing
nursing or midwifery services first
The biggest issues for respondents in Morgan's (2019) study were sensory needs and communication in childbirth – more importantly, the results of how both interact in many autistic profiles.

- The impact of sensory overwhelm – negative rating of 37.74% (strongly disagree and slightly disagree) to:

- – 'Q1 – I felt my sensory needs were considered seriously at the appointments.'

- Similarly negative response (34.54% strongly disagree and slightly disagree) for:

  - – 'Q2 – I felt like I could communicate my needs effectively to the midwife.

This suggests that appointment environments are failing to help facilitate communication, and is pertinent when considering evidence of alternative pain experience.

You make their care and safety your main concern and make sure that their dignity is preserved and their needs are recognised, assessed and responded to

- 'I often found it hard to transition into a state where I could assertively articulate my needs at the right time. Hospital is a difficult and traumatic experience for autistics' (Morgan 2019).

- 'I was not able to express my needs/questions fully, and so therefore just went along with what I was told' (Morgan 2019).

You make sure that those receiving care are treated with respect, that their rights are upheld and that any discriminatory attitudes and behaviours towards those receiving care are challenged

- 'I have not told my health professionals here about my diagnosis, which was made in childhood in the US. I'm gen X and it's common for people my age to hide it in these settings for fear of discrimination' (Morgan 2019).

1 Treat people as individuals and uphold their dignity
Morgan (2019) found:

- 40.95% of respondents disagreeing that they lacked autonomy over being touched by medical professionals ('Q10 – I felt I had consent about how and when I was touched during observations').

- For a population more likely to have suffered trauma, abuse and gender dysmorphic traits, autistic women arguably require more opportunities for consent and bodily autonomy.

- 'Q8 – I knew where to access support after appointments' – 45.37% could not agree they were informed.

- 'Q6 – I knew how to inform the medical practice if I was not happy with my care' – 51.39% could not agree they were informed.

- 'Q5 – I knew I had the right to change midwives if I needed to' – 49.79% could not agree they were informed.

To achieve this, you must:

1.1 TREAT PEOPLE WITH KINDNESS, RESPECT AND COMPASSION

- 'I felt I was looked down on by the staff, I was unsupported and made to feel like I was being over-dramatic' (Morgan 2019).

1.2 MAKE SURE YOU DELIVER THE FUNDAMENTALS OF CARE EFFECTIVELY

- 'Some thought it wasn't a good idea for me to have a baby at all' (Morgan 2019).

1.3 AVOID MAKING ASSUMPTIONS AND RECOGNISE DIVERSITY AND INDIVIDUAL CHOICE

- 'Also, one of my twins was quite ill when he was born, and this doctor kept saying to my husband that I might not be able to cope looking after him. I felt that this doctor didn't understand my needs and autism as a whole!' (Morgan 2019).

1.4 MAKE SURE THAT ANY TREATMENT, ASSISTANCE OR CARE FOR WHICH YOU ARE RESPONSIBLE IS DELIVERED WITHOUT UNDUE DELAY

1.5 RESPECT AND UPHOLD PEOPLE'S HUMAN RIGHTS

'Do not equate Autism with safeguarding risk - we make excellent mothers, but we need systems to work for us otherwise it sends us into a downward spiral that is actually not of our making but entirely as a result of exclusionary environments and systems' (Morgan 2019).

2 Listen to people and respond to their preferences and concerns

To achieve this, you must:

2.1 WORK IN PARTNERSHIP WITH PEOPLE TO MAKE SURE YOU DELIVER CARE EFFECTIVELY

This can mean people having interoceptive differences, particularly in relation to pain, bodily changes and baby movements. Obviously, placenta placement can be checked via ultrasound to address placenta placement factors, but some autistic patients reported feeling kicks differently, less often or more often. Working on an individual level with the patient to identify and attune to these differences in interoception could be incredibly helpful.

- 42.56% autistic women agreed they felt interoceptive, bodily changes during pregnancy sooner (than neurotypical peers or textbook information) (Morgan 2019).

- Alexithymia may be at play so training on this as part of informing an autistic-adapted care plan is essential.

2.2 RECOGNISE AND RESPECT THE CONTRIBUTION THAT PEOPLE CAN MAKE TO THEIR OWN HEALTH AND WELLBEING

This can include taking birth plans seriously and writing them collaboratively if needed. This may include individualised pain scales, language choices or sensory adaptations. Morgan (2019) found that only 14.85% of respondents agreed that they wrote the plan collaboratively with medical professionals involved in their birth.

- 'I felt generally well-informed of what was going on during birth' resulted in only 27.7% women agreeing.

2.3 ENCOURAGE AND EMPOWER PEOPLE TO SHARE IN DECISIONS ABOUT THEIR TREATMENT AND CARE

2.4 RESPECT THE LEVEL TO WHICH PEOPLE RECEIVING CARE WANT TO BE INVOLVED IN DECISIONS ABOUT THEIR OWN HEALTH, WELLBEING AND CARE

2.5 RESPECT, SUPPORT AND DOCUMENT A PERSON'S RIGHT TO ACCEPT OR REFUSE CARE AND TREATMENT

In Morgan (2019), a lack of choice was implied in many interpretations, including consent over examinations, birthing venue, self-advocacy, pain communication, care access and the choice to become a parent. For example:

- 'Some thought it wasn't a good idea for me to have a baby at all.'

- 'I was forced to undergo a parenting assessment before birth.'

And:

- 'Don't touch us without permission and clear explanations. No examinations without clear consent!'

Conversely, some participants reported positive, collaborative relationships with medical staff resulting in more patient-centred outcomes. However, answers recommending good practice observations frequently implied the importance of medical professionals encouraging freedom of choice. For example:

- 'I felt respected in that moment for the individual I was, because she honoured my choices for myself, even though she thought my choice was strange.'

2.6 RECOGNISE WHEN PEOPLE ARE ANXIOUS OR IN DISTRESS AND RESPOND COMPASSIONATELY AND POLITELY

- 'Watch the ones who look like they're friendly and outgoing but then pull the curtains around themselves. They probably need to recharge. Respect that' (Morgan 2019).

- 'My homebirth midwife researched autistic people and autism until she felt able to give the best care. She really went above and beyond' (Morgan 2019).

And:

- 'Health visitor who is retiring soon is lovely. She listened and didn't place preconceptions on me. Instead she asked, so what can I do differently to support you?'

It has been the experience of the authors when speaking on this topic to professionals that they are often receptive and indeed grateful for the infor-mation, feeling it will benefit their practice. The concept of metacognition suggests being aware of what you know and using that information to help you learn and fill any gaps in your skills and knowledge. Often healthcare professionals have such scarce training in autism that their response is that they had no idea, and that this information will help them and in turn help those they support immensely. Following is a recollection of an encounter with a midwife we met with after presenting at PARC London on the topic of autistic birth:

After presenting at the conference, we were approached by a practising midwife from the UK. Emotionally, she told us she had been a practising midwife for 20 years and had never received a moment's training on autism. She said that our presentation had opened her eyes to the vital importance of recognising autistic characteristics and supporting women, and the need for robust training for health professionals. She said that she was now thinking over her caseload in a new light, as someone who practises midwifery within a specialist team supporting vulnerable women from a range of backgrounds.

She recounted one experience with a woman she had been supporting through her pregnancy. It was unclear whether this woman had an autism diagnosis or not, but she said she recognised many of the characteristics and specific issues in her. The woman had become increasingly over-whelmed and distraught and was now at a point in her labour where an emergency caesarean section was required. However, when the anaesthe-tist was to administer the epidural, she was too overloaded to comply. She began to scream and refused to stay still, exclaiming, 'It's not worth it, just get it out of me.' The anaesthetist appeared to make a snap judgement about the woman, thinking she was not putting her baby first.

The midwife said she instinctively knew that this woman was com-pletely overwhelmed. She stopped everything, stepped in, held the woman's hand gently but firmly and told her she could do this, and that they were going to take a breath.

The woman calmed in time and agreed with the administration of the epidural. The midwife, recalling this with tears in her eyes, said, 'I knew the woman was not being difficult. She was the bravest woman I have ever seen in my life.'

Following the conference, the midwife spoke about how she now realised the issues many autistic women may experience and how she would share the information with her team. She added that if she had not pursued attending the conference personally, she may never have gained this insight. It is hoped that the information contained within this book will inspire many more midwives and health professionals to reflect upon their practice and recognise, as this midwife did, the need for individualised care and support.

Creation of a training package for midwives/healthcare professionals

Important note: If anyone discloses that they have thoughts about ending their life, midwives have a duty of care to refer them for appropriate support. Midwives and health professionals are trained to openly listen to women and ascertain the level of risk of harm to themselves or others. For instance, if a woman appears distressed and discloses that they want to end their life, then the appropriate referral would be the ambulance service for immedi-ate referral to a mental health professional at hospital. If the woman has previous poor mental health, she may already be in the care of a perinatal mental health team and so a referral to them could be made urgently too. In the case of a person having suicidal thoughts who says they have no intention at the moment to end their life, an immediate referral to a GP and the perinatal health service could be made. The referral would be the same for those who present with low mood and depression. It is important to explore feelings of anxiety with people as they may be anxious in relation to pregnancy or motherhood, which could be addressed through support or information. For example, some women may fear having blood tests because they do not know what to expect. This could be discussed and practical adaptations could be made to make such tests comfortable. Most areas in the UK have wellbeing and mental health services who would be willing to advise midwives with appropriate advice surrounding referral to other services.

Included here is information on the creation of a proposed training package for midwives/healthcare professionals. It is hoped that the specifics of the autistic birth experience outlined in earlier chapters reinforce the need for such a training package and for such training to be implemented nationally. Table 6.1 summarises the key components of the training, and Table 6.2 outlines a sample seminar for the introductory (bronze) level of training.

Table 6.1 Key components of the training

Recommended duration of training	Dependent on the level of training accessed – see training framework schedule below.
Content of training	A PowerPoint seminar delivered by a knowledgeable trainer to include medical, scientific and historic autism knowledge base before tailoring specifically to maternity care. Resources such as handbooks covering the salient points and examples of visual sensory aids would be beneficial and available to attendees. Content will begin at base 'bronze' level and systematically 'step up' to a more advanced programme.
Delivered by a suitably qualified trainer	Person specification should include someone educated to postgraduate level with a specialism in autism. Ideally, the trainer would embed themselves in the maternity service for at least 2–4 hours prior to delivering the training to suitably tailor the content. Ideally, the content would be developed by or co-produced with autistic women. It is beneficial for the autistic community to have to input into matters concerning them that goes beyond mere tokenism, as per Arnstein's (1969) Ladder of Participation. This will help to ensure training covers all key aspects faced by autistic women.

Who would benefit from this training	Midwives would be the primary target for such training. However, all staff involved in maternity care would benefit, as all may come into contact with the autistic person and influence their experience. This could include switchboard operators, receptionists, nurses, doctors, consultants, surgeons, anaesthetists, health visitors, social workers and other relevant support staff.
Attendee numbers	Dependent on the level of training accessed, as detailed below. At introductory or 'bronze' level, ideally no more than 30 attendees to allow for interaction and discussion during learning. Limiting to smaller attendee numbers allows for more time for reflection and application to practice, as well as more time for questions from attendees and feedback from the trainer throughout.
Cost-effectiveness	Whilst online training is the most cost-effective way to reach a wide number of professionals, it has its limitations, and it can prove difficult to deliver depth and breadth of knowledge, as well as crucial opportunities for activities, engagement and interaction. Incorporating an element of reflective practice under a suitably qualified mentor is shown to be a vital element of professional development in nursing (Caldwell & Grobbel 2013).
Measure of effectiveness	Feedback and evaluation forms completed by the attending professionals after the seminar. Widespread distribution of questionnaires to women in maternity care in the pilot setting prior to and upon completion of the training to quantifiably measure perceived improvement in support. The implementation of in-depth questionnaires and focus groups targeting autistic childbearers, their loved ones and key professionals could further enhance the overall data, providing qualitative feedback as well as quantitative, which could be beneficial in assisting ongoing monitoring and quality control, measuring effectiveness and as justification for wider application.

Outline training package sample seminar plan – introductory level (bronze)

Table 6.2 Seminar plan – autism and maternity care

Background information:	Seminar framework:
To instil a foundation of knowledge of autism, the diagnostic criteria and essential theories. To explore emerging concepts of neurodiversity and autistic voice. To explore the impact on life and the role of intersectionality in societal barriers. To apply this knowledge specifically to healthcare with a further specific focus on maternity care, utilising good practice and professional standards to meet needs, and reinforcing with knowledge-based empathetic care and reasonable adjustments. To investigate some potential issues in pregnancy, birth and the postnatal period with opportunities to reflect and apply to individual professional practice.	• What is autism? An overview of diagnostic criteria and other essential theories • Functioning labels and other terminology • Impact on life, intersectionality and reducing barriers to care • Promoting wellbeing across the wider determinants of health • Sexual health and family planning • Pregnancy support • Adapting the clinical environment • Differences in pain processing and expression • Coexisting conditions and their impact • Facilitating 'safe stims' and coping with sensory challenges • Promoting dignity and autonomy • Why we should think about #MeToo in the birth room • Prior trauma • Person-centred planning • Communication adjustments • Visual supports and their range of uses • Preparing for transition and the importance of continuity of care • Coping with specific challenges in the postnatal period • Supporting carers to ensure their wellbeing
Number of learners: 25–30	**Seminar duration:** 4 hours (5 hours with inclusion of short breaks for coffee and lunch)

Standard resources:

PowerPoint presentation, registration sheet, seminar booklets/links to further information, evaluation sheets, certificates, other resources below

Principal learning outcomes:

• Baseline knowledge of autism
• Impact on life and specifically health(care)
• Best practice examples
• Environmental adjustments

Post-seminar evaluation: evaluation sheets to be issued to all attendees – handbook bringing together trainer's notes, activities, links to further information, etc.

This would be detailed further across a suggested training framework from bronze to platinum:

- **Bronze:** Introductory training for all staff who will have contact with autistic women during maternity care. This will be beneficial for frontline staff in administrative roles as well as health professionals.

- **Silver:** An intermediate level of training which will allow more detailed content and more opportunity to reflect upon implications for practice. Ideal for healthcare professionals who have more interaction than bronze level.

- **Gold:** An in-depth training for all midwives and health professionals who are likely to take a significant role in caring for autistic women.

- **Platinum:** Ideally, in each maternity setting there would also be one autism-specialist midwife, who has undergone platinum-level training – i.e. a longer in-depth course with a smaller attendee limit to enable more opportunity for case study discussions and reflective practice for the midwives, and a 'train the trainer' element which would include facilitation skills to enable them to take on an 'autism champion' role, disseminating their knowledge and upskilling other professionals.

Precedent exists for such specialist midwives. For example, various local health boards have specialist midwives and other maternity professionals for other enhanced needs as below:

- Safeguarding/Child Protection/Domestic Abuse
    - Community midwives receive additional training so they are able to help and support victims of during pregnancy.

- Specialist Midwife for Ethnic Minorities
    - Provides additional assistance to women from minority groups.

- Sure Start/Flying Start
    - Gives additional care and assistance to pregnant teenagers.

- Substance Misuse
    - Available to help women who misuse substances during their pregnancy.

- Maternity Bereavement Specialist

    - Midwives who receive additional training to help you and your family.

(Newcastle upon Tyne Hospitals NHS Foundation Trust 2023; Newry SureStart 2023; Nottingham University Hospitals NHS Trust 2023; Royal College of Midwives 2023; University Hospitals of Morecambe Bay NHS Foundation Trust 2023)

Perinatal mental health teams are an important resource and have been a key focus in the Everyone's Business campaign (Maternal Mental Health Alliance 2018). They may be best placed to be upskilled to provide autism specialist services.

Enhanced training may translate to increased cost, which could prove a deterrent in commissioning, as could the increased time commitment. A health board may also struggle to meet demand with only one or two specialist midwives when sickness, holidays and shift patterns may not correlate with need. This issue may be overcome by building a module as described focusing on autism and related conditions into student midwifery training, leading to a more skilled future workforce. Additionally, such training could be structured to offer CPD points, which may increase its appeal to healthcare professionals and their managers.

Each training level would involve a different duration of training and a different number of maximum attendees:

- Bronze: 4 hours, maximum number of attendees 30

- Silver: 7 hours, maximum number of attendees 30

- Gold: 10 hours, maximum number of attendees 20

- Platinum: 20 hours, maximum number of attendees 10.

Platinum level includes a 'train the trainer' element which will allow fixed-term licensing of organisation course materials and resources included, with the option to refresh and renew at a reduced cost after this period, thus creating specialists in each area who can disseminate their training, creating a greater understanding amongst all relevant staff.

Training and development of resources will likely be a significant investment. However, there is a growing acknowledgement that the NHS needs to change, with a movement towards integrated health and social care. The House of Care model describes a move away from traditional paternalistic reactive medical care to patient partnership and holistic care encompassing all elements of health and wellbeing, suggesting that 'radical redesign of services' with patients at the heart of the process is vital (Coulter, Roberts & Dixon 2013).

The House of Care model encompasses:

- organisational and supporting processes
- engaged informed individuals and carers
- person-centred coordinated care
- health and care professionals – committed professionals committed to partnership working
- all of these 'pillars' to feed into commissioning decisions.

The Kings Fund report on the £3.8 billion Better Care Fund established in 2013 with a 'spend to save' philosophy places emphasis on integration of health and social care and recognises the NHS needs to change to survive, with focus on preventative holistic interventions tailored to individual conditions that fit in with the model of an autistic-specific maternity service (Bennett & Humphries 2014).

Key themes in the development and delivery of the training are:

- co-production
- values-based
- underpinned in learning theory
- reflective practice and continuing professional development
- SMART/prudent use of funds/return on investments (ROI)/ reinforces rather than replicates.

Co-production

Co-production and participatory research is essential in autism research (Stark *et al*. 2021). It is an increasingly held belief that co-production is essential – and successful! – not only research but in development of training, resources, service design and individual care (Chown *et al*. 2017; Kong *et al*. 2019). We refer to Arnstein's Ladder of Participation (1969) which suggests that citizens should be involved in true partnership, being empowered, heard and listened to, rather than being included in decisions about their services, systems and care in a tokenistic fashion.

With this in mind, our opinion is that training packages should *always* be co-produced with autistic/neurodiverse tutors/staff and often delivered by autistic/neurodiverse tutors. This provides the benefit of personal insight, tempered by academic knowledge and balance and the perspective of wider reading and engagement with the local, national and online autistic community. In our professional experience as trainers, evaluations and feedback often comment specifically on the value and power of a tutor/materials with a personal insight of the topic. Gill Phillips (Byrom & Downe 2015) talks about how she has seen the value of involving service users in dementia care – the 'whose shoes' approach – and how this is applicable and valuable in maternity care. Likewise, Havercamp *et al.* (2016) comment upon the values and benefits of inclusion of a panel of autistic people and their family members/carers in training in healthcare.

AASPIRE (2023) has an online toolkit for autistic adults – although based in the US, it is still useful as a starting approach to NHS methods. Its creators, Raymaker and Nicolaidis, regularly publish papers and reflections on how effective and evolving their approach to participatory design for healthcare improvements for autistic adults can be.

Values-based

In addition to the strong belief in co-production that is intrinsic to this proposed training package, there are other values-based aspects to the development:

- **Relativist leaning philosophy (Bloom 2008):** Our ethos is relativist leaning, in that we believe in the value of positivist approaches and quantitative data, but also feel, particularly in relation to autism, that experiences of the world around us are subjective and open to many interpretations based on perspective. Thus we feel strongly that qualitative data brings a depth, richness and unique insight to information and development of materials.

- **Person-centred planning:** We believe strongly in the principles of person-centred care, although we acknowledge they can be difficult to achieve, particularly under funding and time pressures. We feel that services should meet people's needs as appropriately as possible, rather than people having to slot into one-size-fits-all provision. We feel that we should strive to be as bespoke and tailored as we are able within the confines of circumstance in order to secure best outcomes.

- **Active voice in their own care:** We believe that everyone has a right to autonomy, even if independence is not possible. This means an active voice in their own care and decisions over their lives and bodies. Only 12.44% of autistic respondents in Morgan 2019 agreed with the statement 'I felt the medical professionals had time for me when I needed it', and only 12.84% agreed with 'I felt like I had adequate information about who was responsible for my care during my stay'.

- **Basic needs must be met first:** We understand, as Maslow's (1943) Hierarchy of Needs suggests, that basic needs have to be met in a stepped fashion to allow for higher-order activation – thus we feel it is key to ensure a person's basic sensory, social and other needs are met via informed evidence-based practice and reasonable adjustments, to allow them to engage in communication and decision making.

- **Sensitivity in language/terminology:** We endeavour to follow the wishes of the majority of the autistic/disabled community in regard to preferred terminology in all of our seminar materials/resources and when speaking to groups. We realise individual preference may still vary so we respect each person's wishes when interacting on a one-to-one basis. We avoid the use of deficit-based language and aim to be sensitive in both our terminology and our discussion of emotive topics.

Learning theory

We believe all of our materials should have an underpinning in learning theory. This can be a complicated topic but we incorporate elements of anthropology, psychology and education into much of our work. We believe that experience reinforces learning and always incorporates practical activities and opportunities to relate theory to practice in our sessions. We believe learning is valuable not just in the acquisition of skills and knowledge but in team building and strengthening.

We again refer to Arnstein's (1969) Ladder of Participation, (see Table 6.3) this time in a specifically learner-based focus. We believe that the more engaged a participant, the more valuable and expansive a learning environment/opportunity will be. For this reason, our training package framework is structured to allow increasing learner control and empowerment as the levels build.

Table 6.3 Learner participation based on Arnstein's Ladder of Participation concept

Type of participation	Type of involvement	Level of engagement	Examples and advice – autistic community
Manipulation	Directed by staff and tend not to be informed of the issues May be asked to 'rubber stamp' decisions already made by staff	Non-participation	More often seen with big organisations' campaigns May include spokespersons, paid endorsements or outsourcing to non-specialists who happen to share a particular minority identity
Decoration	Indirectly involved in decisions or campaigns but are not fully aware of their rights, their possible involvement or how decisions might affect them	Non-participation	This may be autistic persons not made explicitly aware of the right to attend virtual or in-person policy consultancy meetings
Informing	Community members are merely informed of actions and changes, but their views are not actively sought	Non-participation	Changes to policy are announced once confirmed and are emailed to affected parties in newsletters or social media without participation from affected parties
Consultation	Community members are kept fully informed and encouraged to express their opinions but have little to no impact on decisions	Tokenism	This may be attending virtual or in-person policy consultancy meetings without making it accessible to the autistic voice (e.g. verbal communication, input importance weighted in favour of neurotypical perspective)

Placation	Community members are consulted and informed Learners' views are listened to, to inform the decision-making process, but this does not guarantee any changes learners may have wanted	Tokenism	'A seat at the table but no say on the menu' – participants are invited to join and kept up to date of progression and end results but their input may not have explicit/direct consequences
Partnership	Community members are consulted and informed in decision-making processes Outcomes are the result of negotiations between staff and learners	Tokenism	For example, a supermarket chain announces accessible 'quiet hours' but marketed primarily to parents of autistic children and young people After input from the adult autistic community, the supermarket changes its approach to be inclusive of all ages
Delegated power	Staff still inform the agenda for action, but community members are given responsibilities for managing aspects or any initiatives or programmes that result Decisions are shared with staff	Learner empowerment	A large NHS health board (or clinical commissioning group (CCG)) liaises with previous community activists to take on advocate roles to inform new neurodiversity-affirming support leaflets for local GP and hospital waiting rooms Advocates report back with feedback from the community

Type of participation	Type of involvement	Level of engagement	Examples and advice – autistic community
Learner control	Community members initiate agendas and are given responsibility and power for management of issues and to bring about change Power is delegated to learners, and they are active in designing their education	Learner empowerment	Community members group together, collate their specific skills and expertise to organise a campaign for change, new health initiatives or policy changes, e.g. Maternity Autism Research Group (MARG)

Source: Based on Arnstein's Ladder of Participation (1969)

Table 6.3 can be used as a guide by autistic people and those intending to work with them in participation or collaboratively.

We find this theory further reinforced by Bloom's (1956) taxonomy, where we begin with basic concepts and understanding at our bronze level, steadily increasing learner confidence, control and input, moving steadily upwards, at mid-range, to independently drawing connections and applying gained knowledge to new situations, until, at the highest level, participants have gained the skills to direct their own learning, disseminate their knowledge and upskill others.

We find value in multisensory styles of learning – that is, visual, kinaesthetic, auditory – although we accept there is a lack of clear evidence on the merits of these concepts. We find that mixing styles of learning helps keep the subject interesting, invigorates participants and provides variety, which helps appeal to a diverse range of learners. We feel that visual learning has particular benefit in reinforcing teaching for autistic people, and that the inclusion of movement is important to focus and concentration for autistic people; therefore, interacting with our participants in this way has multiple benefits of engaging learners, reinforcing learning and delivering skills that can be beneficial in engaging with the population we focus our training on.

We find value in innovative styles of pedagogy too, such as pedagogical theatre (Stilman & Beltramo 2019) – based upon Boal's Theatre of the Oppressed (1993) – whereby learners take an active role in the process, which has the benefit of being a novel, memorable and engaging approach.

Reflective practice and continuing professional development

A key theme in the literature of nursing, teaching and other professions is that of reflective practice (Gibbs 1988). We feel that reflective practice offers control over our own learning and evolution of ideas, as well as allowing a clear framework to process both positive and negative events.

We believe it is important to continually update our knowledge, materials and resources in line with the latest scientific/academic research and the views of the autistic and healthcare communities. We aim to pass this 'growth mindset' on to our learners and encourage them to take control of their own continuing professional development. In any field, it is our belief that if you do not continue to update your knowledge, you do a disservice to yourself and others.

Prudent use of funds

SMART goals

SMART goals (Doran 1981) are:

- Specific

- Measurable

- Assignable

- Realistic

- Time-related.

Examination and justification of cost is always an issue in healthcare, where there is a duty to ensure the most prudent use of public funds (Walsh 2016), and the necessity of having SMART goals (Doran 1981) is key. In the current climate of austerity, with an increasingly pressured NHS, justifying a spend on training, particularly when it applies to a specific minority of the population, is essential. Walsh *et al.* (2013) state that this should go beyond 'feasibility' into true cost–benefit analysis.

With this in mind, the proposed training framework has been explored with costs and potential benefits, although pilot training, evaluation and monitoring would be necessary to truly prove the potential feasibility, longevity and benefit of wider implementation. Healthcare reform has been argued to be suffering a need of investment in kindness and compassion before budgetary issues are brought into focus (Youngson 2008).

Why is the cost unavoidable?

Despite multiple constraints, services must provide the best care possible, and legislation means equality cannot be overlooked. The Autism Act 2009 in England states that there must be an autism strategy that provides guidance to the NHS, including planning of relevant services for autistic adults and training of staff who provide these services, and Wales seems set to follow with a new Autism Code of Practice being considered presently that is likely to specifically include appropriate access to healthcare. Legal implications for failures under such legislation, under the Equality Act 2010, Human Rights Act 1998, UN Convention on the Rights of Persons with Disabilities 2006 and the Disability Discrimination Act 1995, can potentially lead to litigation with negative financial implications. Autism has been included in the NHS key priorities, and intrapartum care has also been a topic of much campaigning and consideration in recent years (Maternal Mental Health Alliance 2018). Add to this the additional costs both to the NHS and the general UK economy if negative effects result from traumatic birth, for instance, and the temptation to save funds in the short term on specialist care may prove less than prudent in the long run.

There do not seem to be many alternatives to the proposal – less specialist training perhaps, maybe induction for newly training professionals/midwives that covers a range of disabilities/conditions, which is a good option as far it goes, and should be promoted, but it does not meet the gap in terms of the ageing profession we already have in Wales and the UK as a whole.

It is an option to continue to provide no specialist training on autism, perhaps letting staff interest dictate what they pursue in their own time and at their own cost, or potentially funding conferences and seminars out of a continued professional development budget if one exists. Perhaps the most appealing alternative option would be subscription to an inexpensive or nationally created e-learning module for basic upskilling.

Often the argument is made that if the principles of good practice and person-centred planning are followed, then there is no need for specialist intervention. That may well be true in an ideal world, but the literature shows that currently we are not meeting needs. An overhaul of the whole system might go some way to improving matters, but realistically that is neither a likely nor a timely solution.

The most likely alternative to implementation of training and consultancy is that we continue with the current state of circumstances, where women and their families are faced with dissatisfaction and a lack of appropriate provision to meet their needs. Data from Birthrights found that around a quarter of disabled birthing people had poor or poorer perceived levels of respect from professionals and equally negatively affected healthcare quality compared to their neurotypical peers and 'the majority of disabled mothers felt healthcare professionals did not exhibit appropriate attitudes to their/the patients' disabilities' and 'a minority (19%) of disabled mothers found that despite the omnipresence of the Equality Act 2010 in the UK, reasonable accommodations in perinatal and maternity care services were not made available' (Birthrights 2016).

Return on investment (ROI)/benefits
Ogbonnaya, Tillman & Gonzales (2018) found in a large-scale study of professionals in the NHS – 66,930 employees across 162 organisations – that training had multiple benefits, including team building, enhanced employee wellbeing and patient satisfaction. There could be the beneficial impact of suggested increased staff retention due to increased job satisfaction and engagement.

Who will benefit?
There are potential benefits not only for autistic women but also for their autistic/non-autistic family members/carers, and for autistic family members/carers of non-autistic women. There is also potential benefit for midwives and other healthcare professionals, in that it broadens their knowledge and experience and contributes to their overall professional development. These benefits could aid in career satisfaction and engagement, thus providing potential benefits to health boards in terms of staff retention, engagement and productivity.

Pragmatically, it can be said there is potential political capital in commissioning/committing to enhanced autism knowledge in healthcare. Many in the autistic community have expressed discontentment with services, provision and politics, and a commitment such as this could potentially bring goodwill and enhanced citizen satisfaction.

Spillover effects
Negatively, it is not only financial cost but also the cost of time for staff attendance on training that needs to be considered. In the case of the 'train the trainer' model, licensing of materials would be included for a fixed time period, thus meaning future costs in order to refresh learning

and renew subscription, although this would be less expensive if existing platinum-level staff were still in post.

There is the cost of printing the provided template resources for each woman/family as needed over time, and if nationally developed resources were developed and hosted online, this would have an additional financial and labour cost, although it could allow for women/families to access and print their own materials, so there may be an offset potential in that.

Time spent with each family would likely be enhanced from usual practice, which could have an impact on workload and staff availability.

There is also the potential that a pilot project, including monitoring and evaluation, may uncover other disguised needs and costs.

There is potential to attract professionals to this speciality, which could be positive in terms of autism-specific knowledge, but there is a possibility this will mean drawing staff away from other areas in the NHS where they are needed.

It should also be noted that some professionals in healthcare have come to view mandatory training as a blight on the system, or indeed that it has 'metastasized…like an incurable cancer' (Adhiyaman 2019). It could be argued that inflicting mandatory training on professionals will not only fail to benefit them or their patients but could diminish the overall enthusiasm and engagement of each learner group as a whole.

In respect of autistic women/families, there could be wider economic benefits of more positive healthcare experiences, such as better health and improved infant bonding, which could have a positive effect on child development. It could also mean greater opportunity to work for families, which boosts the economy and could reduce welfare benefit dependency. With improved health, there may also be less reliance on health services, mental or physical, in the long term.

Finally, resources developed and distributed could be useful for groups other than the intended target group – including those with ID/LD, mental health conditions such as anxiety, or for those for whom English is a second language.

Nature of the costs

The difficulty with the nature of the costs involved in implementing the training nationally is a large upfront expense to health boards, both in terms of funds and staff time commitment. However, if some of the projected benefits around staff retention and user health prove to be viable, these costs are likely to be offset and recouped.

Importance of reinforcement, not replication

It is important that the training and materials complement and reinforce rather than replicate existing provision and resources – which is why during development a preliminary scope of the existing literature and resources is always carried out and a 'links to further information' resource is always provided, detailing potential further relevant reading and resources. It is also important to recognise that sometimes beneficial information, e-learning and resources have been developed to meet the needs of other user groups that are still helpful and relevant for those supporting autistic women and their families.

Need for targeted resources

For a pregnant autistic woman, who may have already internalised a huge number of deficit-based messages throughout her life, the emotional labour of trawling the internet for quality, robust, sensitive information can be a monumental task – it could be hugely difficult at times to face yet more negative and damaging information whilst looking for answers, guidance and support.

There are often freely available resources and information for varying issues that can be utilised and signposted, such as advice and resources for sexual abuse survivors or easy-read versions of documents created for other target groups that may be beneficial or adaptable. By virtue of the 'train the trainer' model, we would be equipping staff with the knowledge and skills to begin to identify and adapt such materials on a case-by-case basis.

There is more and more information available for women during pregnancy and birth with the advent and expansion of technology, social media and the online world, which can be beneficial for autistic women – look for websites and apps that provide visuals, clear information and suggested timelines of pregnancy and birth. Checklists and guides on how to prepare and what to expect may be helpful, and apps to manage all sorts of things, including pregnancy progression week by week to timing contractions, to mindfulness, to tracking newborn sleep and feeding, may also be beneficial.

An essential message to include is that approaches, interventions, strategies and resources may have to be tailored not just to the differentiated needs of autistic women as a group, but also to each autistic woman's unique and individual needs, which may also differ.

Practical advice and strategies

- The quality and continuity of care is vital. Elements of good practice such as respecting birth plans and providing clear information may be even more imperative.

- Underlying knowledge and sensitive use of language is also paramount; equipping healthcare professionals with information about sensitive use of language around autism, gender, sexuality, mental health, disability, etc. is important, including the use of identity-first, non-deficit-based language.

Language around autism

Research suggests that the majority of autistic people prefer to be referred to as autistic rather than a person with autism – this marks a shift from the promotion of 'person-first' language, particularly in professional settings. That being said, personal preference may vary – and it is key to respect the values and wishes of the person and their loved ones in one-to-one situations. Potentially helpful in navigating language and terminology is the policy we use at Autside (Autside Education and Training 2023), and which will apply to our created training package for healthcare professionals, included below:

Use of language – Our policy at Autside

Team Autside have given consideration to our use of language, understanding that it evokes strong responses and should be sensitive to the Autistic community. We acknowledge that there will be 'no one size fits all' policy that will fit with everyone's wishes, as we know there is much debate around preferred terminology.

We have decided on the use of identity first language rather than person first language, i.e. 'Autistic' rather than 'has Autism', after considering recent research, the views of the Autistic community, and of our Autistic tutors and Director.

All our materials will reflect this decision, and we will continually strive to ensure our ethos remains in line with the wishes of the community. We will of course endeavour to use personal preference in individual instances where this preference may differ.

We also feel strongly that the language and terminology used around Autism and disability should be respectful and wherever possible focus on difference rather than impairment. This would include:

- Not using terms such as illness or disease in reference to Autism

- Using terminology such as predominant neurotype, neuro-typical, or non-autistic rather than 'healthy' or 'normal'

- Avoiding the use of phrases such as 'suffering from Autism'

- Avoiding the use of descriptions such as 'treatment' or 'cure' in respect of Autism interventions

We acknowledge that a lot of the content we deliver can be of a sensitive nature and carries a significant potential emotional impact. All of our trainers endeavour to be sensitive in the discussion and delivery of this content. We understand that language is fluid and continually evolving, and thus remain engaged with the Autistic community, valuing your continued input and feedback.

'Nothing about us without us.'

Disability is not a dirty word

Terminology and language around disability is an emotive topic. Whilst there are many varying opinions, it is our view that we should not shy away from the use of the word 'disabled'. However, using terms such as 'confined to a wheelchair' should be avoided, with many wheelchair users expressing that rather than being 'trapped or confined', their wheelchair use allows them additional freedoms.

Supporting autistic people with gender identity differences

Gender identity differences occur where a person experiences discomfort or distress because there's a mismatch between their biological sex and gender identity. This is separate from sexual orientation.

- **Gender identity:** How you see yourself.

- **Sex assigned at birth:** What the medical community labels you.

- **Gender attribution:** How your gender is perceived by others.

- **Gender expression:** How you want to present your gender.

Gender expression can be conscious or subconscious. Your gender may be expressed through your actions, what you wear, your hairstyle, make-up or other elements of your appearance as well as the pronouns you use.

Gender pronouns are words or phrases that describe the gender of a person. Preferred pronouns are the gender pronouns a person feels most comfortable using. These may be based on gender identity or expression and can change/fluctuate.

Terminology around gender

We may hear lots of different terms used and it might be difficult to understand something we may not have ever felt or experienced ourselves. Here are some of the terms that might be used when referring to gender variances:

- **Cisgender (cis):** Someone who identifies with the gender they were assigned at birth due to biological sex.

- **Transgender (trans man/masc, trans woman):** Transgender is an umbrella term to describe someone whose gender is not the same as the sex they were assigned at birth.

- **Gender fluid:** A person whose gender identity fluctuates across the gender spectrum.

- **Non-binary (enby):** A person who does not identify with a strictly male or female binary gender.

- **Gender questioning:** Someone who is in the process of questioning or exploring their gender identity.

- **Demigender (demigirl/demiboy):** Feeling a partial but not full connection to a particular gender identity.

- **Genderqueer:** Someone who may identify as being both male and female or falling outside these categories.

- **Gender non-conforming:** Someone who does not conform to 'traditional' or 'established' gender norms.

There is sometimes confusion around sexuality and gender, and it is important to reinforce that they are two distinct concepts. Sexual orientation – for example, heterosexual, homosexual, bisexual, asexual – is about who you are sexually or romantically attracted to. There is often an interplay between gender and sexuality, but this is complex and should not be assumed.

Much like gender identity, sexual orientation is not always a binary. The Kinsey Scale (Kinsey Institute 2023) has its limitations but was a pioneering tool to explore human sexuality as a spectrum and has since birthed more tools such as the Klein Sexuality Grid (Autistic Empire 2023).

Dos and Don'ts around gender identity

Avoid:

- birth names/dead names (the birth name of a transgender person who has changed their name)

- misgendering

- asking for or showing pictures/descriptions of how they used to look

- insensitive/inappropriate questions.

Instead:

- listen

- believe them – we may find it hard to understand if we have not experienced anything similar but it is important for the person to feel validated

- ask for preferred pronouns and use them

- ask them what help and support they need.

You may get it wrong – and if you do, apologise but without making a huge deal out of it.

Gender exploration versus gender transition

Someone may explore their gender identity without deciding to transition. In other cases, they may explore their gender for some time and then decide to transition. There are many ways in which someone can affirm their gender and 'transition', and which of these a person pursues is determined by personal choice but may be impacted by other factors such as safety, access to healthcare, finances and more.

Gender variance, autism and the birth experience

As you may anticipate, pregnancy and birth can be a particularly emotive time for those experiencing gender differences. It may contribute to increased feelings of dysmorphia, and chestfeeding may also introduce a need for specialised care to meet individual needs in an empathetic, sensitive way.

Person-centred

Remember, everything we do should draw on useful information we learn about the wider autistic community, but should always be applied uniquely to each individual. As Dr Stephen Shore said, 'If you've met one autistic person, you've met one autistic person' (Flannery & Wisner-Carlson 2020).

Creating a person-centred autism passport

Not all autistic people will find a health passport useful as many of the ones in circulation use language and visual methods to support people with a learning disability. However, examples of supportive and individualised adjustments which can be made within the healthcare setting are available (e.g. Henry 2023). Individualised care plans can be downloaded and used in their entirety or they can be used to gain ideas for adjustments which enable accessible maternity care (Henry 2022).

Wellbeing indicators and screening for postnatal depression

Birth trauma and prior existing mental health conditions are indicators for developing PND. The support autistic women require in the postnatal period may differ, and traditional interventions for PND may need to be tailored/adjusted. We also need to be mindful of how we assess for PND, too – for example, midwifery notes on 'lots of visitors today *smiley face*' as indicators for mental wellbeing may not be a good measurement for autistic/neurodivergent people with differing social needs and wants.

Managing and assessing pain

Pain assessment and management need to be adjusted in autistic women, with consideration given to communication aids and alternative measurements of pain. Recent research has suggested heart rate monitoring (Failla *et al.* 2017) and some studies are beginning to advocate for the use of Fitbit-type wearable tracker devices to monitor heart rate and blood pressure as indicators of distress (Koo *et al.* 2018). Summers *et al.* (2017) advocated for continuing development of tools to assess pain in ASD, suggesting consideration be given to 'physiological indicators and neuroimaging techniques'.

Fertility and infant loss

We need to be aware that autistic people may respond to and express feelings of grief and loss differently and may need help to process what has happened in a more tangible way. Autistic people may experience delayed grief or work through the stages differently – and although we might not appear upset in the expected way or say the expected things, that does not mean we are not hurt or grieving.

Autistic women report their sensory sensitivity means they recognise signs of pregnancy earlier and more intensely:

> Many autistic mothers have shared that they became very aware of their internal body state and knew things about their pregnancy before the textbooks said they should…
>
> Autistic processing can be very different to the average person's, and some may not process what has happened immediately or even within the weeks and months that follow the loss. (Tommy's 2022)

In addition, it is the same sensory sensitivity that creates a barrier to accessing care when experiencing a pregnancy loss, as in many instances this would mean making a phone call, being able to describe pain and attending a hospital with a busy waiting room (Grant 2022). Another issue identified is around the language used by health professionals in relation to pregnancy loss. Autistic people have reported that they did not understand they were experiencing a loss or that their baby had died because vague language was used to inform them. It is essential, therefore, that any findings are shared concisely, and understanding must be confirmed.

Resources and tailored information

It is important to note that any resources used should ideally be tailored to the specific autistic person. There is always a risk of 'unintended consequences' partially due to literal interpretation by an autistic person who is supplied with ambiguous, confusing information, or information or visuals that are not best suited to their developmental level, learning style or processing ability. For some autistic people, overly simplified information will seem condescending and not offer the level of insight and knowledge they require, while for others simplification is vital. Thus, it is key to have a robust profile of the person you are supporting and to tailor the resources you provide accordingly. This section will provide some example resources and factsheets, which will be available to download and edit as needed for individual patients.

Data from Morgan (2019) indicates the following:

- Overall, poor patient satisfaction was reported with the transition to parenting at home. This is generally represented by 8.02% agreeing with the statement:

    – 'Q29 – I felt like I was offered long-term postpartum support to meet my needs.'

- More specifically, when asked about distinct aspects of care related to a common co-occurring issue in autistic women, mental health-care planning was similarly rated negatively. Only 17.26% of autistic women agreed with the statement:

    – 'Q25 – I felt like my postpartum (post-birth) mental health needs were taken seriously.'

- Only 6.82% agreed with the statement:

    – 'Q27 – I felt like my co-occurring conditions (or other long-term conditions) received adequate care and planning.'

Although participants were not required to disclose the nature of the mental health conditions, the seriousness is imporant since the early parenthood period needs vigilance on mental health for most women, but particularly for a community that has such higher incidences.

It is useful for healthcare providers to tailor information for autistic people and to provide visuals, either written, illustrated or ideally a combination of both for autistic people to keep and process in their own time. This could include a range of potential factsheets/easy-read visuals on topics such as:

- Family planning:

    – contraception

    – intimacy and autism (including sensory differences)

    – healthy relationship dynamics

    – consent

- unexpected pregnancy – options and links (including morning-after pill, abortion, adoption, etc.)
- planning for a baby
- fertility issues
- 'Do I want a second child/more children?'
- Pregnancy:
  - 'Could I be pregnant?'
  - what to expect – body, emotions, etc.
  - what to expect – healthcare journey, standard appointments/scans/healthcare professionals involved
  - making an autism passport
  - anxiety during pregnancy (spotting, etc.)
  - pregnancy and gender identity
  - supporting siblings
  - autistic partners/loved ones
  - self-care during pregnancy
  - communication with professionals
  - reasonable adjustments/risk assessments at work.
- Preparing for birth:
  - choosing a health setting
  - choosing a birth partner, supporter or doula
  - making a birth plan/relaying wishes to supporter(s)
  - packing a hospital bag
  - tips for loved ones – how to support in the lead-up to the birth
  - what happens during labour and birth – water breaking, contractions, etc.
  - pain relief options

- prenatal classes
- Braxton-Hicks contractions
- coexisting conditions and medications.

- Preparing for baby:
  - 'What equipment will I need?'
  - choosing the best options.

- Impact of Covid-19.

- During birth:
  - communicating and consent
  - managing anxiety
  - processing, expressing and coping with pain
  - unexpected changes
  - vaginal birth
  - interventions
  - C-section.

- After birth:
  - recovery
  - dealing with trauma.

- Adjusting to parenthood:
  - coping with change and implementing new routines
  - postnatal depression
  - energy accounting/spoons/social battery (see Chapter 7)
  - sensory issues
  - family dynamics – house rules/family contract
  - extra help and support (direct payments, mental health, accessing both autistic and new parent communities)
  - breast or chestfeeding

- bottle feeding.
- As the baby grows:
  - childcare
  - work
  - finances
  - weaning
  - milestones
  - health visitor
  - socialisation.
- Energy management and managing expectations (optimistic realism?):
  - social battery
  - spoons
  - energy accounting.

Other resources could include 'What's that?' sheets, with explanations of terminology/shorthand with visuals such as 'fluttering', crowning, sweep, dilation, etc. or what to expect during each stage – including physical and emotional symptoms, infant development, advice during labour, explanations of stages, sensations and so on.

It can also be useful for appointment letters to include visuals such as maps/photographs of the buildings, names, pictures and roles of the professionals and what to expect during each appointment.

At my first scan, the letter I received prior suggested I drink water before attending. It was unclear how much, so I drank one small bottle around 500ml. This clearly was not enough as the scan technician berated me for not drinking enough and sent me back to the (very crowded/noisy) waiting room with instructions to drink as much as I could and NOT to go to the toilet until they called me back in. By the time I was called back in an hour or so later, I was in agony having drunk a lot of water and with my anxiety having ratcheted up to alarming levels, unhelped by the busy clinical environment and my intense need to urinate. During my scan, my distress was clearly overlooked, with the technician laughing that I now had drunk far too much and would be back and forth to the loo all day. I was also berated for having a body piercing in my belly button, being told it could damage the equipment and I should have removed it before the appointment. Despite being apologetic and explaining I had not realised, and offering to remove it immediately, I was told not to bother, but made to feel awful for my oversight.

By the time of my second (20-week) scan, I was determined not to experience this again, so I vowed to drink as much water as I could prior to my partner picking me up for the appointment. I drank nearly two litres of water in a short window of time, and was terrified when my vision started to dim and black out, Luckily, I vomited up the water, and only later did I learn of the dangers of drinking a large amount of water in a short space of time. When I told the scan technician about this experience later, she laughed and said they didn't even really need my bladder to be full at this stage in pregnancy in any case as the baby was bigger now. I found all of these experiences humiliating, painful and anxiety provoking, and they were all avoidable with the provision of clear, understandable information.

Emma

Simple tips that might seem obvious to other people would have been so helpful to me. After having several stitches post-labour, I was experiencing a lot of pain vaginally, especially when urinating. I could only bear urinating if I took the somewhat unhygienic step of getting into a shallow bath to do so. However, I was absolutely exhausted, from the trauma of birth, adjusting to motherhood and the effect on my other health conditions/disabilities, and as such I could not manage climbing in and out of the bath so regularly. I began to reduce the amount of fluid I drank in the hope I would need the toilet less. This obviously impacted both my health and my milk supply. Only days later on noticing how dark my urine sample was did the midwife realise this issue, and advised me to pour a jug of lukewarm water over myself as I urinated, or press a warm soaked flannel to myself to reduce the pain. I could have kicked myself – it seemed so obvious but just hadn't occurred to me and caused so many more problems than it needed to. I have a habit of making things harder than they need to be!

Emma

CHAPTER 7

Practical Strategies and Information

In this chapter, we will bring together all the topics discussed in earlier chapters and consider the impact this can have on professional practice, including standards of care such as the NMC code. Hayley will also present findings from her original research and Emma will present her proposed training plan for healthcare professionals.

- Recognising difficulties in pregnancy

- Recognising difficulties during labour/birth

- Recognising potential difficulties adjusting to parenthood

- Recovering from birth

- Coexisting conditions

- Understanding behaviour

- Low-arousal approach

- Coping with meltdowns and shutdowns

- Visual supports and alternative communication

- Preparation, planning, familiarisation, reassurance

- Supporting executive functioning

- Fostering independence and autonomy

- Setting goals the SMART way

- Sensory supports and environmental adjustments

- Emotional toolkit

- Building self-esteem

- Supporting successful socialisation

- Use of technology

- Involving carers/supporters

- Safe spaces

- Intense interests

- Respecting personal objects

- Energy management

- Strategies for demand avoidance

- Supporting those who are undiagnosed but suspected/seeking an autism diagnostic assessment

- Some 'top tips' for maternity/healthcare professionals

- Autistic advocacy: accessible rights during pregnancy and motherhood

If you have serious concerns about the wellbeing of any patient, such as severe anxiety/depression, self-harming behaviour, suicidal ideation or an eating disorder, please refer them on to professionals who can give more targeted help.

Recognising difficulties in pregnancy

A number of the difficulties encountered by the autistic birthing person during this time are likely to be related to difficulties in the following areas: difficulties with interoception and sensory overwhelm from the bodily changes of pregnancy, difficulty with hormones affecting mood, feelings of isolation from inherent societal or communication barriers, difficulty with executive function (particularly in terms of booking and attending appointments), difficulty with feeling heard and communicating needs in appointments, difficulty with anticipating changes that giving birth will mean – whether in relation to bodily changes, or in terms of practical differences in life with a new baby.

In addition, autistic women may find being touched challenging, which makes scans, blood pressure measurements and abdominal palpations difficult. Prior discussions with women are essential to gauge their level of difficulty with being touched so questions can be asked about how they can be supported. It may simply mean that the women are provided with a list of routine checks that take place at an antenatal appointment and information about why they are performed, which can prepare women to have their blood pressure taken before their appointment. A pregnancy communication plan may be useful to prepare women for the care they may encounter during pregnancy, labour, birth and the postnatal period (Henry 2022).

Recognising difficulties during labour/birth

Some of the difficulties an autistic person is more likely to face during labour and birth may be centred around the following: interoceptive difficulties relating to pain processing, body temperature or other bodily changes, difficulties or differences in communicating needs around this bodily information (e.g. absent or different pain communication), alexithymia resulting in one sense being confused for another (e.g. cold instead of anxiety or vice versa), masking or fawning resulting in a difficulty in recognising and/or communicating true needs.

In addition, the labour and birth experience can change very quickly and go from a calm, controlled environment to one where change is necessary and communication is inhibited by the need to act quickly. For example, women often arrive in the birthing environment with a birth plan which the midwives read and implement and can create a calm, controlled environment. However, if any deviations from the plan are recommended, for example a vaginal examination is indicated earlier than planned because there are signs of labour progression, then the midwife would communicate this in a concise way to share situational information. This situation may be difficult for autistic women due to needing more time to process such information and they may become anxious around changes. Such feelings may impede a woman's ability to hear the information, process what has been suggested and share her thoughts. It is essential, therefore, for midwives to understand such difficulties and perhaps discuss the possibility of care plans changing during labour and birth in the antenatal period so that women can almost plan for such events through implementing communication alternatives. It may help for information to be given to the birth partner who can support the woman to communicate and give consent to any changes to care.

Recognising potential difficulties adjusting to parenthood

> After my child's birth I just desperately wanted to go home, rest, recover…
> But my home didn't exist any more, my whole universe had imploded,
> irrevocably changed – and I couldn't catch my breath…
>
> *Emma*

- Routine:
  - Our routine is often not just altered but utterly decimated with the arrival of a mini human.
  - Coping with this change can be particularly challenging for an autistic parent.
  - We can try to introduce new routines, but these do not always go to plan, which can be frustrating.
  - It can be hard not just emotionally but physically and cognitively to adapt to a new way of life and a different day-to-day experience.

- Anxiety:
  - General anxiety as well as anxiety about parenthood, and our child's safety, etc.
  - Feeling we have no control over our environment or routine can be really difficult.
  - Trigger points that are difficult for most parents can be unbearably anxiety-inducing for some autistic people – first day at nursery/school, trips away, first sleepover, etc.

- Sleep disruption:
  - Our sleep can be massively disrupted by a new arrival. Sometimes this persists throughout childhood.
  - Exhaustion can make it even more difficult to regulate our emotions.
  - Exhaustion can also make our sensory differences even more hypersensitive and difficult to cope with.

- – Executive functioning is affected by a lack of sleep, making daily tasks really challenging.

- Lack of 'downtime':

  - – Downtime is important for everyone, and a lack of downtime can be challenging for everyone. However, this replenishment time is absolutely vital for autistic people to self-regulate and recover from things like sensory overload.

  - – Unfortunately, downtime can become seemingly impossible for parents – whether it is a new baby, a curious toddler or a rebellious teen, finding time to rest can be challenging.

  - – This can lead to shutdowns, meltdowns and burnouts for the autistic parent.

  - – There is no easy answer to coping with the reduced downtime, but things like using sensory interventions/adjustments, being conscious of your energy levels and where you can 'save' and 'spend', and utilising any support you do have can help.

  - – If there is another parent, then sometimes 'tag teaming' is the only way to manage and ensure you both get some time alone to rest.

  - – Otherwise, support networks with other parents where you 'trade' playdates so the kids can socialise can offer some pro-tected time. Or accessing direct payments/respite may allow that time if possible.

- Sensory overload (page 140).

- Uncertainty, confusion, emotional regulation (pages 107 and 126).

- Executive functioning (page 50).

- Impact on relationships (pages 55 and 67).

- Social support (page 100).

- Stigma, judgement, intervention (page 113).

- Overwhelming visitors, house calls and a 'new social world':

  - – From the early days and weeks after birth, parenthood intro-duces us to a whole new social world. After birth we are often inundated with visitors and wellwishers which, while it is lovely to feel cared about, can be intensely overwhelming. Even letting people into our 'safe space' can prove a challenge, which in some cases begins in those first days and weeks but often emerges in more varied ways throughout our child's life.

- We may struggle with scenarios such as parent and baby or parent and toddler groups.

- We may find elements of school life such as sports days, coffee meetings, school plays or other events challenging.

- Our children may wish to invite friends over for playdates, meals or sleepovers. They may enjoy extracurricular activities such as sport, crafts, etc. which include a level of expected interaction between parents. There may be birthday parties to organise or attend.

- There may be things we previously avoided but now find it increasingly difficult to keep up with social demands and expectations, as well as navigating the social 'politics' in the school yard or at other groups.

How can we help ourselves navigate this new world?

- Sensory aids – for example, Calmer earbuds are well reviewed and, unlike noise-cancelling headphones which may be impractical for parents who need to listen out for their babies or children, they reduce noise whilst still allowing you to be aware of sounds in your environment.

- Emotional tools and anxiety management (page 206).

- Self-care (pages 42 and 216).

- Seek support (page 199).

- Preparation (page 200).

- Executive functioning aids, routines, visuals and organisation (page 202).

- Shortcuts and hacks are OK! We are here to tell you that you do not need to prepare organic vegan baby food from scratch – unless you want and are able to. If you feed your family convenience food at times, so be it. There are lots of shortcuts out there like steam vegetable bags, microwave rices, pre-chopped fruit and vegetables and so on. This doesn't make you lazy! We understand finances play a role here, however, in being able to afford such things but they can make life easier and for some of us might be vitally beneficial helpers.

- Energy accounting (pages 186–187).

- Communication (page 148).

- Link with other autistic parents (page 220).

Recovering from birth
Differences in parenting style and mixed neurotype parenting
Autistic parents will face specific challenges and bring specific strengths in raising children, but often we 'do things differently'.

We may be judged for our parenting methods as they might fall outside of 'the norm', and we may bond and show affection differently.

> I think a lot more about parenting than a lot of the other people I know.
>
> *Kirsten Hurley*

> I think I had a pretty extensive 'outline' in my mind of how I wanted to parent before we even began trying to conceive. I considered the 'big questions' and 'key moments' and had planned for them, even rehearsed them in my head before our child even existed!
>
> *Emma*

We provide support for neurotypical parents of autistic children, but there is no similar support for autistic parents of neurotypical children who are also facing the challenges of mixed-neurotype parenting. This is an area that is currently massively overlooked and under-served, as neurodivergent parents may have the same struggles understanding and communicating with their neurotypical child as neurotypical parents do when their child is neurodivergent.

Coexisting conditions
As autistic people are highly likely to have one or more coexisting conditions, a holistic view is vital. This should take into account how autism may affect experience but also other conditions may also impact – for example,

trauma responses may lead to increased anxiety or sensory sensitivity, fibromyalgia could increase pain, eating disorders could be triggered by weight gain or bodily changes during pregnancy, and so on.

> I am just me – a whole person with my own unique personality, rather than a set of symptoms which can be easily recognised to one of my 'conditions'. (Mind 2015, p.23)

Understanding behaviour

We can only truly tackle behaviours that are problematic by taking the time to understand the function of the behaviour. We need to recognise that many factors will impact on someone's outward behaviour and that these may not all be immediately visible or recognisable. Likewise, people may struggle to identify and understand their own behaviour, too. It takes time, patience and effort to truly understand each person's stressors and anxiety levels.

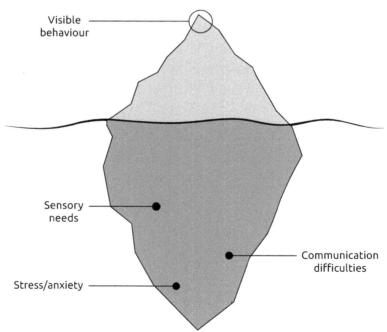

ICEBERG
Understanding behaviour tool

Visible behaviour is often just the 'tip of the iceberg' – it is vital to uncover and resolve the underlying functions of behaviour.

Figure 7.1 The tip of the iceberg

A favourite tool is the iceberg (see Figure 7.1), which suggests visible behaviour is only ever the 'tip of the iceberg' and is actually a result of many underlying drivers beneath the surface, such as:

- underlying unmet needs
- difficulties in communication
- frustration
- sensory overload
- emotional regulation difficulties
- gaps in understanding, skills/knowledge
- developmental factors
- anxiety
- struggling to complete tasks/process information
- pain/health issues
- impulse control difficulties.

We tend to use the unofficial term 'Sherlocking', which really means being the detective. We need to use tools such as the iceberg, the STAR chart:

- Setting
- Trigger
- Action
- Result

or the ABCs:

- Antecedent
- Behaviour
- Consequences

to help us figure out what the underlying function of behaviour is, because only then can we truly support someone and meet their needs.

Reframe our perspective

It can be helpful not only to those you support but to you as professionals to reframe your perspective:

- 'They are so difficult' becomes 'They are having such a difficult time'.

- 'They want attention' becomes 'They need connection and reciprocity'.

- 'Their anger is out of control' becomes 'They need help to identify, understand and regulate their emotions'.

When we recognise that a lot of behaviour we perceive as challenging is in response to anxiety, overload, emotional dysregulation or communication difficulties, for example, we respond and react differently.

This empathy and understanding can lead to longer-term or more effective solutions for everyone!

Low-arousal approach

A low-arousal approach is often advocated whilst supporting autistic people. Key elements of this approach include:

- being non-confrontational

- having realistic expectations and avoiding overload

- communicating clearly and calmly.

A low-arousal approach works best if used consistently, but it is not an immediate 'cure all'. It isn't the natural way to react in stressful situations, but we can take note of and alter our behaviour with conscious effort.

Coping with meltdowns and shutdowns
Adapting our communication during meltdowns and shutdowns

- Make less eye contact.

- Keep your voice at a lower pitch and volume.

- Use fewer words and simple gestures or signs.

- Make fewer requests.

- Use slower, controlled breathing.

- Slow down your movements, relax your posture and don't tower above the person.

- Keep your distance and avoid touching.

- Remove any audience.

- Repeat to yourself, 'I can pretend to be calm'!

- Go at the person's pace.

Put yourself 'in their shoes'

A lot of anxiety and phobias can be irrational or catastrophised to seemingly epic proportions, and as such it can be easy to dismiss these as silly – but remember, they are very real indeed to the person experiencing them, and this will only make them feel worse, and less likely to share how they are feeling and what they are thinking in the future.

We hear a lot of people say things like 'pull yourself together' or 'snap out of it'; this is ultimately not helpful to someone dealing with depression, anxiety or intrusive thoughts.

Be honest and factual

Another thing that is tempting is to make promises we can't possibly keep in the face of anxiety.

For example, if someone is facing a recurrent fear of death, it can be tempting to promise that we aren't going to die for a very long time. People will realise this isn't something you can promise, and it may only serve to make their anxiety worse, or make them less likely to trust any future reassurances you give them.

There are ways to reassure people whilst still being honest. For example, instead of outright promising you are not going to die anytime soon, you can ask them how many people do they know who have died? What ages were those people? How many of their friends have lost parents? And then explain this is because it is not likely. Also tell them what the plan is in the unlikely event they do die. It may be a difficult discussion to have, but it can provide necessary reassurance.

Visual supports and alternative communication

Recent research suggests autistic people socialise effectively with each other (Crompton *et al.* 2020; Kaufman 2020). Autistic people often place value on different methods of communication, and often benefit from visual aids with a mix of text and illustrations. Again, this is a good example of what benefits autistic people actually being helpful for everyone, as many of us benefit from visual supports in our daily lives, such as road signs, menus and maps.

Visuals are a complex area and there are many methods available, which could include supports such as:

- communication 'shortcuts' – cut-and-paste phrases and visual supports, which are also helpful for other conditions and where English is a second language

- wristbands or lanyards

- communication fans

- apps/software or alternative/augmentative communication (AAC)

- visual schedules

- pain communication alternatives such as a communication fan – where is the pain, what is the type of pain (throbbing, stabbing, etc.), how severe (based on numbers or colours)

- communication bands/badges

- help cards

- prompt cards

- phone or watch with pre-programmed phrases or images, handy apps or assistive language software.

We need to be aware of common communication mishaps, where we may assume that someone either didn't hear, won't comply or is being rude, but this is often not the case.

It can be helpful to avoid sarcasm, idioms and metaphors unless you know the person well or they display clear understanding of these concepts, as there can be literal interpretation that leads to confusion and/or unintended consequences.

The way we phrase a question can make a difference. Questions beginning 'Can you...?' may be answered 'Yes' but then the person doesn't actually do the aforementioned thing – with a literal interpretation, this answer is perfectly appropriate, as the question phrasing only asked if they 'was able to' do the said thing, without actually requesting they do it.

Preparation, planning, familiarisation, reassurance

All of us need some support to manage our lives. Being autistic in a world not designed for your neurotype can be unpredictable, chaotic and confusing.

Structure helps provide a lifeline in a sea of unknowns – some certainty which can be an absolute necessity to cling on to.

Autistic adults often need help to know:

- **what** is going to happen

- **when** it's going to happen

- **who** is going to be there

- **where** it is happening

- **how** and **how long** for

- **how they will know** when it's finished.

Preparation and planning can reduce anxiety. A lot of autistic people need routine and sameness for comfort and security. Although it is good to try to build in elements of flexibility wherever possible, routine and planning can provide a much-needed lifeline to cling to for an anxious autistic person.

Visual supports can be extremely effective in reducing anxiety and supporting executive functioning. There are many visual supports you can use, such as:

- Social Stories™ (Gray 2000)

- visual timetables/schedules

- 'now, next, later'

- timers

- tracking a journey with Google Maps/satnav

- cards

- bracelets

- traffic light symbols
- calendars/diaries
- weekly/monthly/yearly planners
- step-by-step task overviews
- decision trees
- reward systems
- checklists
- mind maps
- labels.

We can support preparation and planning in a range of ways, including via:

- role play
- examples/Social Stories (Gray 2000)/videos
- video tours
- other familiarisation techniques.

Supporting executive functioning

In order to support someone effectively, we must meet basic needs first as per Maslow's Hierarchy of Needs. We can then build a strong foundation of executive function skills in three areas:

- environment
- relationships
- activities.

It is vital we individualise our approach considering age, ability, interests, strengths, difficulties and goals.

Fostering independence and autonomy

When supporting to embed new skills and knowledge:

- Gradually increase complexity/challenge.

- Remember there are often many facets to what seem like simple tasks.

- Giving an autistic person clear, visual, step-by-step instructions can reduce the overall demand they may be facing.

- Remember that independence may take longer or arrive in a different order, at different times, but development never stops.

- Simple visual schedules can assist with a person learning to complete chores and tasks, both around the home and for self-care and hygiene, as well as embedding new skills needed to care for newborns.

- Offering an option to check off, rip off (Velcro) or earn a reward/point adds motivation to complete the task and can boost self-esteem.

- Sometimes, beginning with a visual schedule and 'backward chaining', we can guide a person through the process until they are familiar and can gradually increase independent skills.

Think of it as building a staircase of skills step by step. Often, by breaking tasks down into chunks, we can reduce a huge amount of executive function burden. Remember, executive function does not correlate with intelligence.

It is also vital to ensure we provide safe spaces, practise patience, compassion, kindness and empathy, and 'nudge not nag' by using reminders, prompts and praise. We can further support executive function by embracing intense interests and harnessing hyperfocus, and reducing processing demand by making time external, thinking about whether they know how long each activity/task lasts. We can provide early warnings, such as:

- timer

- time tracker

- sand or egg timer

- 'five more minutes'

- 'last time' or 'finished'

- traffic lights.

Role play and modelling, practising or acting out scenarios, watching video modelling and engaging in conversations and example stories can prove helpful.

We also need to ensure we are meeting physical needs. There may be an increased need for movement/movement breaks, so consider easy ways to introduce bursts of physicality where appropriate, such as physical games, star jumps, clapping or gentle yoga where safe to do so.

Sensory needs also need to be considered, such as encouraging safe stimming and providing appropriate sensory interventions.

Ensure that the person's 'fuel' is topped up – remember that interoceptive differences mean an autistic person may not feel the need to eat or drink, but the need may still be underlying, so prompt for regular snacks/drinks.

Engaging in puzzles and games can be calming and can focus the mind, and for some autistic people, sorting and categorising can be calming – for example, sorting beads by colour and shape calms me by making me feel a sense of order, control and things having their right place.

Think about how you can optimise the birthing or clinical environment for an autistic person. There may be limits to what you can do here, but simple adjustments can make a big difference.

Setting goals the SMART way

- Break goals into chunks.

- Big goals – what smaller steps will I need to achieve them?

- It is important to think about how much is too much – an overloaded person loses executive function.

Embedding essential life skills, like knowing how to dispose of different items, when to discard food, toiletries or medications past their use-by date can make a big difference.

Modelling behaviour – modelling daily tasks, showing them how you make decisions about what to let go or how you complete chores and home organisation gradually – is helpful.

See it, do it alongside, do it independently…

Sensory supports and environmental adjustments
Creating an individual sensory profile or 'passport'

- It is important **to build up a picture** of where an individual is hyper- and/or hyposensitive.

- We can use this to **inform others** of what they may find difficult and what they might need/enjoy.

- We can also use it to look for **healthy stimulatory activities** or to identify where we need to try to reduce environmental or other demands.

- Occupational therapists will often complete a **sensory assessment** and use this to inform a **sensory programme or 'diet'** to meet the individual's needs.

- This kind of **individualised or 'person-centred'** planning is vital in autism because it is often so varied and complex.

Sensory aids

- Fidget toys:

  - Putty, fidget cubes, clothes tags, fabric, elastic bands, tangle toys.

- Chewelry.

- Deep pressure:

  - Either through weighted interventions such as blankets, lap pads, wrist/ankle weights or through 'squeezes' or firm massage. Deep pressure is a therapy where touch or weight is used to help people who have sensory sensitivity. It uses pressure via touch to help someone who may need proprioceptive input to desensitise or cope with anxiety or overload. This can be achieved by squeezes (Temple Grandin made a squeeze machine), a squeeze vest, firm hugs or massage; or weight – weighted vest, blanket or lap pad. Tighter clothing is also an option in other circumstances, but this is advised against during pregnancy and after childbirth.

- Body brushing – different types of brush can have different effects, such as desensitisation of the top layer of skin or calming/regulatory:

- – This can aid in desensitisation to tactile dysfunction and improve tolerance to clothes.

- – It can be a calming therapy.

- – There are a variety of brushes available, including surgical brushes, body brushes, facial brushes, hair brushes/Tangle Teezers.

- – The type of brush and how much pressure is applied and for how long will vary for every individual and can fluctuate.

- Complementary therapies such as aromatherapy.

'Stimming'

The term 'stimming' is short for self-stimulatory behaviour, also known as self-regulatory behaviour. It is a repetitive movement or sound that provides sensory input. It can help autistic people manage anxiety, cope in difficult environments and manage sensory overload and can be a necessary and even joyful experience.

While it is important to allow autistic people the freedom to stim sometimes, stims can be harmful or undesirable, such as where they cause injury to the person. In these cases, we should look for ways to redirect the stims. We should never expect to stop a behaviour without replacement, as this could increase anxiety, meltdowns or shutdowns, and lead to the development of increasingly harmful behaviours.

It is key that we work on embracing self-stimulatory or regulatory behaviours, finding safe stims that are calming and recognising that stims can also be joyful and pleasurable. This can be difficult for some autistic people who have over time learned to suppress stims either subconsciously, via feedback from society or via interventions such as ABA.

Emotional toolkit

An emotional toolkit contains a range of coping mechanisms, self-care skills and anxiety management strategies. This can help us navigate everyday life, express our needs, wants and emotions, and cope with stress, aiding our overall wellbeing. Effective management of stress is vital to avoid overload, where the brain circuits required for executive function are disrupted, triggering impulsive 'act now, think later' behaviour. These kinds of emotional tools are beneficial to anyone, autistic or not, in today's busy world.

This toolkit may include:

- thinking tools: to test our thoughts

- comfort tools: for feeling safe and, well, comfortable!

- social tools: to combat loneliness

- emotional literacy tools: to help us identify and express our feelings

- relaxation tools: to feel calm and manage anxiety

- physical tools: for wellbeing and energy

- self-care tools: for maintaining our overall wellbeing and equilibrium.

Thinking tools
Testing our thoughts

This is about supporting us to test our logic and to regulate anxious catastrophizing thoughts. We may need help to put things into context, to evaluate the likelihood of anxiety-driven scenarios, to develop critical thinking skills and to scale the importance of items.

Cognitive behavioural therapy (CBT) model

Cognitive behavioural therapy (CBT) is a talking therapy that focuses on how your thoughts, feelings and actions impact each other, while introducing a range of coping strategies for different issues. For some time CBT has been controversial in its application for autistic people. However, in recent years research has expanded into adapting the existing CBT models for better results when working with autistic people. Even if an autistic person does not wish to engage fully in CBT, the underpinning model may still be helpful for them. The model suggests that our thoughts and feelings and behaviours are intrinsically linked and impact each other in a circular fashion – what we think affects what we feel and do, what we feel affects how we think and act and how we act affects how we feel.

Redirection/perspective shifting

Autistic people often 'catastrophise'. It may help to work through and gently help to 'test' their thought process. What's the worst that can happen? If the worst happens, what will I do? What is the best that could happen?

Think about using 'contingency maps', which branch into two or more options, showing potential outcomes/consequences for each decision, rather than traditional visuals that follow one path. This will depend on the individual.

Comfort tools
Comfort bags/boxes
These contain favourite things, photographs and things that make us feel good.

Calming echolalia

> During my labour, one of the only things that somewhat calmed me was to repeat a simple song from a sitcom, over and over. I liked the way the words felt leaving my mouth and the rhythm of it, the frivolity of the tune and lyrics. The familiarity of it helped me to draw upon the feelings of safety and comfort I had felt on the many occasions my partner and I had watched the show at home together and it was one of the only things keeping me regulated when I was feeling almost completely overwhelmed.
>
> *Emma*

Social tools
Social tools can include a range of strategies designed to help build meaningful activities and combat loneliness and isolation, such as Social Stories™ (Gray 2000), which can help to gradually learn the 'secret social rules' (e.g. etiquette in various situations; communication building; learning about complexities such as metaphors and idioms, which can be a small thing that has the potential to cause substantial misunderstandings in social situations), or exploring personalities and relationships via books, television shows and movies and discussing the scenarios, feelings, actions, outcomes and alternatives.

Emotional literacy tools
There are a wide range of emotional literacy tools which could prove helpful, such as:

- **Wheel of emotions:** This is a visual that illustrates core or primary emotions at its centre, expanding into more nuanced emotions towards its outer edge. It can be a useful tool to help identify and 'narrow down' what we are feeling. There are many wheel of emotions resources available online.

- **Somatic emotions wheel:** This builds upon the wheel of emotions in a way that may be of particular benefit to autistic people (and those with alexithymia or other conditions that may impact emotional literacy) by connecting specific emotions to commonly linked sensations in the body. A full overview of the tool and additional information and resources are available at the website of its creator, Lindsay Braman: https://lindsaybraman.com/emotion-sensation-feeling-wheel.

- **Emotional thermometers and scales of emotions:** These provide visual ways for us to help 'measure' our emotion/problem and modulate our response appropriately. There are many free resources based on these concepts available online.

- **Pin badges:** Pin badges with emotional or mood thermometers are available to purchase online and can help the person to think through and scale their emotion and have the added benefit of visually communicating their emotion/mood to others.

- **Blob trees:** Visual resources which portray human 'blob' figures in various poses and situations. for example standing proud at the top of the tree, falling or sitting alone on a branch. They are designed to help draw out and explore emotions by connecting with the 'blob' figure the person is drawn to, as well as discussing emotions more widely by exploring the feelings of each blob character.

Relaxation tools
Mindfulness

Mindfulness takes practice – it's not an easy thing to master. It's easy to give up and think it's not working for us, but it's not an instant process. ADHD and autistic 'busy brains' can complicate the exercise too, but it is worth practising.

Not every visualisation will work for everyone – try different visualisations until you find the right one for you. For example, visualisations of lying in the grass could make someone scared of bugs uncomfortable, or visualisations of floating in water could make someone who cannot swim uneasy.

Tap into good memories if you can. For example, my child is calmed down when I talk them through swimming with dolphins. I quietly and calmly describe the feel of the water, the smell of the air, the squeeze of the wetsuit, etc., and it often works extremely well.

Alternatively you could focus on a specific memory of sensations such as Emily Swiatek's suggestion of a chocolate meditation where she focuses on a specific pleasant experience with all your senses step by step. See NHS Leicestershire Partnership (2023) for more ideas.

Autonomic sensory meridian response (ASMR)

Gaining popularity, ASMR is a bit like Marmite – you either love it or you hate it! But for many autistic people, it has been hugely positive. It focuses in on specific visual and auditory inputs which have been shown to have a physiological effect in a percentage of the population and can prove calming, regulating and satisfying for many. There are many videos available, ranging from simple soap carving to people chewing to virtual optician appointments! Like any other technique, it's trial and error to see if it works for you and which examples work best. Some of my favourites are candle carving and cookie decorating videos!

Grounding

This technique is useful in averting panic, is quick and easy to implement in a range of environments and is designed to 'ground' you and reorient you in your environment.

Take a deep breath and then list:

- five things I can see

- four things I can hear

- three things I can feel

- two things I can smell

- one thing I can taste.

Tapping

Tapping is an anxiety management technique which works by tapping pressure points on the body; it is also known as somatic stimulation. The idea is that tapping can help regulate emotions and calm the nervous system. In the case of autistic people, it can also be a useful sensory input which helps disrupt or block overload. It can help ground us quickly in almost any situation as it is easy to employ, requires no equipment and can be discreetly carried out even in public areas. It can also help us process more deeply rooted traumas over time. An added benefit is that in moments of panic, emotional distress or overload, tapping can work quickly, within minutes. There are specialists who can advise and support people to use tapping effectively, but it is also easily employed by following simple steps:

- Tap your wrist with your opposite hand.

- If needed, say aloud the emotion, worry or memory that is causing stress or anxiety while you tap.

- You can use tapping on other areas of the body such as the top of your head or just above your collarbone. There are many articles online which explain tapping in more detail.

Other anxiety management tools

Anxiety management tools are varied and plentiful and may include art therapy or journaling. Thinking tools such as reimagining outcomes in a positive way, and focussing on the good things to encourage positive thinking and distract from fears, anxiety and catastrophising are also key. (See 'Self-care tools' below for specific ideas.)

Physical tools

Physical tools include exercise, getting out into nature and ensuring we keep ourselves hydrated and 'fuelled' with the right nutrition. That said, it is vital not to add pressure or guilt to a person who is struggling with their physical health, diet and exercise.

Self-care tools

These could include:

- a self-esteem bucket – the idea that we all have individual buckets that contain our self-esteem, which we can fill with positive things, but which gets damaged by negative things/feedback causing our self-esteem to 'leak' or diminish. For autistic people, it can be a constant battle to top up the bucket while the world 'pokes holes' into it.

- talking to yourself as if you are your friend

- positive affirmations

- three good things – this is a simple technique to encourage reflection and positive thinking. It involves saying out loud, to others or even to yourself, three good things that have happened that day or that week. I encourage the families I work with to make this part of their routine either daily or weekly, as it serves as a reminder when things seem negative that there are good things to be grateful for. The teens I work with embraced this concept really enthusiastically and it has helped them communicate, connect and find positives.

- rose exercise – I expand on the three good things concept by utilising the 'rose exercise' which I came across online. I wanted to retain the element of communication and positivity but also felt it was important to allow for expression of frustrations or worries. The idea is that you express how you are feeling in four ways:

  - the flower: something good that has happened

  - the thorn: something bad that has happened, or a worry

  - the bud: something you are looking forward to

  - the gardener: someone who has supported you.

  This exercise was a really useful tool for our emotional toolkits, as it helped with identifying and expressing emotions, sharing problems and worries, and focusing on the good things and the nurturing people around us. Again, I suggest making this part of the daily or weekly routine.

Positive affirmations may sound clichéd, but combating anxiety with positive affirmations can be helpful.

Writing a note to yourself can be a subconscious reinforcement of positive thinking. Using a quote or statement that resonates with you, whether speaking it aloud or reading it regularly, can be helpful.

Building self-esteem

Autistic people often have challenges with self-esteem.

Self-worth can inform our relationship choices – feeling bad about yourself can mean you accept negative treatment you feel you deserve or maintain toxic relationships just to have company. Filling and protecting a person's 'self-esteem bucket' is vital. It is also important that, in cases of vulnerability, we reinforce what is acceptable behaviour, what being a good friend or partner involves and how to 'balance the scales' in relationships so people do not get exploited.

In order to build and protect self-esteem, we need to understand potential challenges to self-esteem for autistic people, which may include:

- negative feedback

- anxiety and catastrophising

- 'getting things wrong'

- perfectionism

- feeling of not 'fitting in' and issues with self-identity

- being overly shielded

- feeling they have little or no control over their life

- feeling everyone is 'against them'

- difficulties with emotional regulation or executive functioning

- always feeling at fault – when it could be entirely unrelated to them

- stigma/lack of understanding

- feeling isolated and/or being bullied or teased.

Supporting successful socialisation
Potential difficulties in socialising and relationships

- Autistic people have difficulty with social rules, which can lead to them learning one way to do things and struggling to be flexible about this.

- Understanding the social hierarchy can be hard.

- Extremes – extrovert/introvert, dominant/submissive.

- Autistic people who are able to mask or camouflage some of their difficulties say it is exhausting – like doing maths all day – basically trying to make logic of something that isn't logical = intellect over intuition.

- The teen years can be the most difficult time of life for many people, autistic or not, and this often leads to anyone different being excluded socially.

- The teen years are also a time of great change, physically, socially, emotionally, hormonally, and often there is a big transition in education too – this can mean complete overload, making socialising even more difficult.

How much is too much?

Some people might love spending lots of time with others, some a bit, others hardly any. Some might like to have lots of different friends, some might like to keep just a special few. There are no hard and fast rules on the right or wrong amount of socialising, just ensuring the individual has the opportunities they want and need in order to socialise safely and happily and avoid isolation and loneliness.

Sometimes our expectations or the expectations of others will differ drastically from what an autistic person can manage socially. Autistic people might have very different social needs to what is expected. They might like more time alone and fewer activities, and might be happy with a small core group of friends. Often autistic people have a reduced social battery that needs lots more recharge time, so it's important not to project expectations of the 'normal' amount of socialisation.

Pacing can be useful here, using tools such as:

- social battery[1]

- spoons[2]

- energy accounting.[3]

Being with the right people

Meeting new people and/or making friends can sometimes be difficult for autistic people. Some of us are great at making friends – but maintaining friendships might be the difficult part...

---

[1] The term social battery describes the amount of energy one has for socialising. See Villines (2023).

[2] Spoon theory describes the amount of available energy you have, measured in 'spoons'. See McCann (2021).

[3] Energy accounting, created by Maja Toudal and Tony Attwood, is a tool to help manage our energy levels. See McKay (2020).

I often think of friendships as flowers lined up on a windowsill – taking a lot of care that at times I can't provide due to my limited social battery – so I say all my friends are cactuses! Happy for me to pop in and water them when I have the 'spoons' to do so…

Emma

Circles of trust

Concepts such as the circles of trust (Figure 7.2) can help autistic people explore where they feel safest and 'most themselves' and where they feel more compelled to mask. It can also help them to develop skills that make socialisation easier and reduce their vulnerability to exploitation.

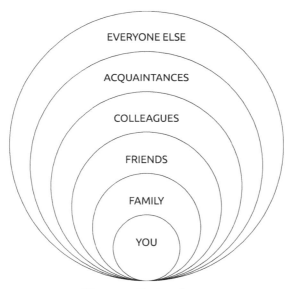

Figure 7.2 Circles of trust

Stock responses

For certain interactions, stock responses can be learned and can be helpful – particularly if an autistic person knows a situation is or will be too draining or stressful for them. This can help them exit or avoid the situation tactfully. Phrases might include:

- Please excuse me.

- I need a break.

- I need help.

215

- Thank you but I have plans.

- I will have to check.

- Can I get back to you on that?

It can also be useful to have stock responses about being autistic and how this impacts them that they can use to explain to others.

Equipping with social skills safely

There are some social skills we can teach, and some we cannot.

When equipping autistic people with information about the world and the social environment, we have to carefully balance providing information and coping skills whilst not encouraging constant masking. It is important to think about what is really important – for example, forcing eye contact is uncomfortable, and can mean loss of concentration on the conversation.

Everyone is different – generally speaking, humans, their thoughts, feelings, emotions and actions are unpredictable and often illogical – so 'teaching' a set of rules is never going to fit every scenario or every person.

Use of technology

Technology can be hugely beneficial for autistic people and has a myriad of uses, including:

- visual supports and modelling behaviour

- calendars, planners, reminders, journals

- relaxation, self-care and emotional expression

- monitoring internal/emotional state (Fitbits)

- learning, literacy, numeracy, science

- gaming: puzzles, brain training, strategy, fast-paced, decision-making games, Minecraft, Lumosity

- productivity: Pomodoro (a time management method to break work into intervals)

- communication and interaction: Proloquo2Go (an augmentative and alternative communication app)

- programming emergency contacts and health information into one's phone

- navigation apps, 360-degree tours and building plans to familiarise ourselves and help us find our way around

- use of apps in establishing routines, forming healthy habits and identifying patterns of behaviour with potentially positive or negative outcomes (on mood, sleep, diet, etc.). Wearable fitness devices such as Fitbits, Apple watches or similar can help with tracking our overall health, wellbeing and mood and identifying which factors impact these positively and negatively; they could also aid in identifying patterns and triggers for overload over time

- apps to aid in communicating emotions.

Alternative/augmentative communication (AAC) are devices or software that allow for a different method of communication. This is hugely beneficial for those who are minimally verbal or reactively mute. These are available as specialist dedicated devices or software/apps for smartphones, tablets, etc. with tools for planning, preparing and organising, such as mind mapping.

Time management

Keeping track of time has never been easier, with our smartphones, smartwatches/fitness trackers and other devices always on hand.

This is hugely beneficial for neurodivergent people who can struggle to keep track of time – and it's great to have digital, customisable options for reading and processing the time too, such as different clock styles.

Many devices also have the ability to set timers, both stopwatch and countdown options – which can be used to:

- time study time

- count down to school or appointments

- time activities

- time chores

- use as a timer for cooking.

All of these can be useful for supporting executive function. This can be particularly beneficial for keeping track of appointments, vitamins, food and water intake, etc. during pregnancy. During birth, timers can help with contractions. For parenthood, when implementing a whole new routine with a newborn, timers and reminders can be more than helpful – they can be essential. They can help with feeding schedules, sleep patterns, bath times, etc., which some parents may find hugely beneficial.

Alarms/reminders
Most devices have the functionality to set alarms that can be:

- single instance alarms

- repeated daily

- repeated weekly.

Some wearable fitness devices include smart wake functionality which aims to help you wake feeling more refreshed – which could potentially help your cognitive function right from the start of each day.

Scheduling
Use your computer, phone, tablet or smartwatch to control your schedule, set reminders and stay focused and organised, as well as supporting structure, routine and time management using apps such as iCalendar, Google Calendar, Outlook or Teamup.

Games and puzzles
Games and puzzles play an important role in strengthening executive function (and other skills!) – and they can be fun too!

- **Fast-paced action games:** Strengthen coordination/dexterity, prioritising, decision making

- **Strategy:** Sims games and role-playing games (RPGs) teach planning, prioritising, consequences and adapting to change

- **Puzzles and memory:** 'Brain training', jigsaws, Sudoku, crosswords, logic games and 'match the cards' flex our working memory, prioritising and decision making

- **Multiplayer games:** Help with turn taking, coping with our emotions and impulse control.

Managing money

Managing finances can be difficult for anyone but if you add in the complexities of autism, ADHD or other neurodivergent or mental health conditions, it can sometimes feel overwhelming or even impossible. Technology can also play a really important role in managing our money. Utilising banking apps can make our lives easier in tracking our income and expenses and allow us to make payments easily. Apps like Monzo can help us budget and allocate money to spend or save in different pots, such as holiday, clothing, house deposit, etc.

There are also apps that assist in making monthly budgets of income and expenditure, which can be helpful.

Health and wellbeing

Technology can help with our overall wellbeing by helping us understand our bodies better. We can track the impact of diet/nutrition, sleep, movement and other health metrics and how they intersect with and affect each other, and set small achievable goals that help us practise self-care.

Travel and transport

Finding our way around, on foot, public or private transport.

- Timetables, purchasing e-tickets, navigation apps, 360-degree tours and building plans can all help to familiarise ourselves and help us find our way around.

- Even accessing images online when visiting a new location can help reduce anxiety and help us pinpoint the location we are looking for.

- For those with coexisting conditions, many destinations now have online accessibility guides which help to let us know where there is wheelchair access and other useful information.

- Even being able to access the menu online for a restaurant, for example, can be a huge benefit to autistic people and their families!

There is some suggestion that data collected by wearable fitness devices can indicate when autistic people are becoming stressed, agitated or frustrated. This could serve as an 'early warning' of overload – enabling us to employ sensory interventions and movement to distract, calm and meet undetected sensory needs. It could also help to identify triggers and build up a picture of what raises and lowers our anxiety levels over time.

Mindfulness and tech

- Mini mindfulness and breathe reminders on Fitbit.

- Various mindfulness sessions online or via apps like Calm or Headspace – Headspace even has programmes of sessions available via Netflix.

- Can set daily/weekly goals to achieve.

- Logging mindfulness sessions to see the impact they have.

Tech and music

If timers make an autistic person anxious, why not try using Spotify/iTunes/Apple Music/Amazon Music/Vevo/YouTube to use a song or playlist as a countdown instead?

Music can also be calming/regulating, which can help executive function by reducing anxiety and aiding focus. It can also be a great way to express how we are feeling in an alternative way, which many autistic people find helpful.

Tech can be vital for autistic people: having our tech with us can act like a 'security blanket'. Many people, autistic or not, say they would be lost without their phone! For autistic people, the reassurance it provides to have coping mechanisms, contacts, and a way to access information and listen to music or play a game is invaluable in so many situations.

Online socialisation

Autistic people often thrive by finding community in forums, support groups, blogs or other social media outlets. There are many signposts for support and camaraderie to be found in neuro-affirming language and ethos alike.

Involving carers/supporters

It is often extremely valuable where possible to include loved ones in the process when supporting autistic people. They can often provide a wealth of information and understanding of the person's specific profile, characteristics, strengths and support needs, and may be able to alert you to any potential triggers for overload.

It is also important as other family members may have additional support needs as we know there are strong genetic links with autism and related conditions. There is also the added benefit of potentially reducing trauma responses in partners/supporters if they feel informed and included in the process. Often carers have been helping to advocate for the person for a long time and know them best, so they may be able to help with techniques that may work or be inappropriate.

Partners can feel helpless, ignored and overlooked during the birth process – and this can lead to trauma. For plans/strategies to work, you need everyone 'on board', and consistency across environments can be key to success, so carers are intrinsic!

Safe spaces

It is key that we create safe spaces for autistic people to think about, prepare for and experience pregnancy, birth and parenthood. This means ensuring their needs are met and that the environment and the discourse within the space is not triggering to them. Mainstream parent and baby/toddler groups may be difficult for neurodivergent parents to access due to anxiety, social differences and sensory overload. Likewise, support groups for parents of autistic children may be triggering with negative discourse around autism, which can be hurtful, and the issues faced may be different for individual neurodivergent parents. This is not always the case, I have certainly made extremely close bonds and true friends for life in some of my forays into autism support groups for parents – and it may be that you meet other undiagnosed neurodivergent parents with whom you can form mutual support and understanding. It is a risk for autistic people entering these groups and facing the unknown though, and that needs to be recognised and mitigated.

Intense interests

Speaking at the NAS #AutismWomen Conference in 2018, Carly Jones said, 'Special interests save lives.'

Monotropism is a cognitive theory that is believed to be central to autistic thinking. It can cause us to focus our attention on a small number of intense interests at any time, meanting that we tend to miss things outside of this attention tunnel.

Intense interests can be not only beneficial but vital to autistic people, not to mention a great source of joy in many cases. They can aid self-esteem, communication and interaction, and often they are instrumental in autistic people feeling they have found their place in the world. They can truly provide a place of safety, security and comfort.

Therefore valuing them and understanding their role is vital, although we may need to set clear boundaries to keep them from becoming all-encompassing.

One good example of using intense interests in managing anxiety and depression is how I use the Harry Potter series of books and movies.

Their author, J.K. Rowling, has a history of depression, and she weaves this experience into her books.

There are two examples you can try from these books as good metaphors to tackle anxiety and panic.

Dementors are black-cloaked, demon-like creatures that guard the wizarding prison, Azkaban. They are blind, but they can sense and feed on positive feelings, draining their victim's happiness. The only way to vanquish a dementor is to conjure a 'Patronus', a kind of shield that appears in a silvery mist in form of an animal. You must gather your most happy thoughts and memories, and fill the Patronus with them, giving it the power to overcome the despair and hopelessness the Dementors make you feel. This 'charm' can help children and adults to visualise themselves overcoming their fear. They can visualise the fear and imagine the patronus dispersing it until it disappears.

Boggarts are shapeshifting creatures that take on the form of your greatest fear. For example, if you are terrified of spiders, a boggart would appear as a spider. The spell to overcome a boggart is 'Riddikulus', which adds some funny, novelty element to the fear, making it ridiculous and therefore less frightening. In the example of the spider, in the books/movies, the spell caused the spider to wear roller-skates, hopelessly slipping and sliding around. Or in the case of Professor Snape, he becomes less frightening in a dramatic ladies' hat and clothes! It is possible to use this technique as a visualisation to overcome fears, negative thoughts and even nightmares. It can be expanded upon – for example, recounting a dream but changing the ending to something funny, or positive.

Emma

Respecting personal objects

This is of course important for any person you are supporting, but there are several reasons autistic people may have an especially strong attachment to objects/belongings; as such, they can be very protective over them and anxious about them being touched or moved.

Object permanence means knowing that an object still exists, even if it is hidden. It requires the ability to form a mental representation of the object.

Object personification is when a person attributes human characteristics, thoughts, feelings and values to inanimate objects.

Research is scant as yet, but there seems to be suggestion this may be a factor for some autistic people.

> My partner says I can 'pixarise' anything – pennies even!
>
> *Emma*

Associative memory is defined as the ability to learn and remember the relationship between unrelated items. Autistic people can have strong associative memories related to an object, and make connections that others may not make.

Some people may feel that without the object they will no longer have the memory – which can make parting with all sorts of items very difficult. Even bodily fluids or hair/nails for some – so having a baby inside you for nine months and then that disappearing...

Autistic people may also collect items that seem to have little value to others. This might be leaves, rocks, shredded paper, food wrappers – and it is possible this could have a sensory function for them.

Energy management

Pacing is a vital skill for people with chronic conditions, in order to effectively manage our energy and maintain wellbeing.

There are several tools we can use to help us do this:

- social 'battery'

- spoon theory

- energy accounting.

They essentially help us build a record to find our baseline and activity 'costs'.

Strategies for demand avoidance

For demand-avoidant people, traditional autism approaches may be ineffective at best and exacerbate difficulties at worst. The rules, structure and strict adherence to routines that are often beneficial for autistic people may have a negative effect in demand-avoidant profile management. Therefore, while some renowned autism management strategies can be adapted to good effect (e.g. visual supports), differing strategies may be necessary and helpful in the management of extreme demand avoidance (EDA).

Key principles

As with autism management more generally, it is important to be person-centred in our approach. Indeed, this is likely to be ever more vital in those with a demand avoidant profile due to the complexity of their profiles and need for differentiated strategies.

Functional assessments that explore the individual's strengths and needs as well as potential 'trigger points' can be useful in creating a holistic, tailored support plan, where we should focus the majority of the strategies on being proactive rather than reactive.

PANDA (PDA Society acronym)

The PDA Society has developed a PANDA acronym to suggest five key strategies for supporting those with demand avoidant profiles:

- picking battles
- anxiety management
- negotiation and collaboration
- disguise and manage demands
- adaptation.

Consistency staff/keyworker

Characteristics of the ideal person to work with individuals with EDA include:

- ability to build a relationship of warmth and trust

- a good sense of humour

- ability to stay calm and neutral

- flexibility

- creativity

- resilience

- ability to think on their feet

- ability to show sympathy and empathy

- ability to self-reflect and stay regulated.

It is particularly key to avoid over-dependence in people with EDA by ensuring you have a consistent group of staff working with the individual, rather than one specific person. There can be a social intensity characteristic to the condition that can cause people with EDA to become hyper-focused on specific individuals, sometimes beyond a point that is healthy for either the person with EDA or the person they are focussed on. This also means that if the specific person is not available at a given time for any reason, this could lead to emotional overload, resulting in meltdown/shutdown.

Managing expectations
This includes managing the expectations of the person with the demand-avoidant profile and managing the expectations of professionals.
   Keep in mind:

- Every interaction is a two-way process.

- Set clear and agreed upon priorities.

- Adjust demands according to level of tolerance.

- Build realistic goals and positive experiences gradually.

- Implement a low-arousal approach.

Anxiety versus tolerance dials
It is important to be flexible and insightful and able to recognise when demands can be increased and when they should be reduced.
   As the anxiety levels of a person with EDA increase, the level of demands

expected of them should decrease – the supporter's dial should always be working in the opposite direction to that of the person with EDA.

Sensory considerations

Individuals with demand-avoidant profiles often have sensory differences, as expected in autistic people.

They may appear very 'hyper' as if 'driven by a motor' with an intense need to 'check' the sensory environment.

The intense anxiety they are experiencing increases this hypervigilance and sensitivity to sensory information to overwhelming levels.

> Idleness is a demand – it's intolerable. I have to be doing SOMETHING.
>
> *Sally Cat*

A creative approach

Being creative and using a range of strategies is key when engaging with people with demand-avoidant profiles. Indeed, switching the methods and strategies used can be key to ensuring the person does not come to 'see through' a particular method.

- Humour can be a very effective strategy at diffusing situations.

- Use areas of interest to engage.

- Build on strengths.

- Use imagination and role play.

- Novelty and spontaneity can work very well.

Communication techniques

How we successfully use communication/language can be quite different for those with an EDA profile:

- Being spontaneous, silly and inventive and 'mixing up' our communication can prove effective in engaging those with an EDA profile.

- Remember, those with EDA profiles often use language effectively but may have lower receptive language ability, so check understanding/allow processing time, as in traditional autism management.

- Use collaboration/collusion techniques – 'What is our mission today?' Be an ally rather than an 'enemy' or a 'boss'.

- Use the person's interests – using characters or objects can depersonalise demands and appeal to the sense of novelty in EDA.

- Humour can distract/lower anxiety – be prepared to make fun of yourself.

- Use of indirect communication methods such as Post-it notes, recorded messages or text message can prove useful – be prepared to switch methods to keep it interesting!

Illusion of choice

This strategy is simple to implement and can boost sense of agency/empowerment by offering choices. This offers a sense of control, thus reducing the extreme demand-avoidant reaction, whilst still achieving the necessary goal.

Offer a choice of two options where both options are suitable:

- This jumper or this cardigan today?

- Would you like an apple or a banana?

Keep the choices minimal to avoid overwhelm – two or three options are ideal for most people, although this is discretionary on a person-by-person basis.

Affirmation instead of praise

- Remember that direct praise can be perceived as a demand.

- Praise can feel pressuring – if they did well this time, you will expect the same or better next time and the time after.

- Indirect praise can be successful (e.g. 'I like how those two colours go together' rather than 'Wow, you're a great artist').

- Regular affirmation is still important, but this can be best achieved by taking an interest in what the person with EDA is doing, or listening to them talking, and showing you value and respect them with your time and actions.

Indirect demands

- Posing demands/questions indirectly may be beneficial when interacting with/supporting those with an EDA profile.

- Use of a character or object to engage with the individual might be helpful.

- Use of technology, including video modelling or AAC devices, could work, too.

- Talk out loud – 'I wish someone knew how to do this'.

If a direct request is part of a normal conversation, it's easier for me to cooperate with. If it feels a gentle question mixed in with a friendly chat, it is much easier than having an instruction. (Fidler & Christie 2017)

Use of visual supports in demand-avoidant profiles

Visual supports are often extremely effective interventions in the management of autism, as discussed earlier – but they often need adaptation for use with those with demand-avoidant profiles.

In demand-avoidant profiles, empowerment is of the utmost importance – for example, involving the person in creating daily visual routines, use of contingency maps instead of traditional visual schedules, or multiple choice feelings boards.

It is essential that visuals are used in a flexible and non-confrontational way and that the person feels they do not add a demand but rather they are a collaboration between the supporter and the individual.

Contingency maps are particularly beneficial because they:

- are indirect

- are visual

- show consequences

- offer options.

Supporting those who are undiagnosed but suspected/seeking an autism diagnostic assessment

The following are ways in which common autistic characteristics may present. This is not an exhaustive list, and everyone may present somewhat differently based on a variety of factors. This may be of use in identifying potential autistic characteristics in someone receiving care, which could help in identifying the best support; however, we would not suggest midwives are best placed to broach the topic of potential autistic characteristics with someone in their care unless the subject is raised by that person, in which case directing them to the below list may help them in recognising signs in themselves and gathering evidence to make a self-referral or approach their GP, mental health provider or local autism team for a referral/assessment. It is worth noting that a family history of autism/neurodivergence may be an indicator for a higher likelihood of autism.

Social interaction/communication

- May find it hard to approach others.

- May find eye contact uncomfortable or unnatural.

- May have to pay a lot of attention to the gestures and body language of others to decipher their meaning.

- May need to concentrate on their own body language in order to 'fit in'.

- May seem to 'space out' in a conversation.

- May find it difficult to initiate conversations.

- May struggle to instinctively follow the flow of a conversation and tell when it is their turn to talk.

- May interrupt others.

- May dominate a conversation (often unintentionally).

- May become easily bored if conversation is on a topic that doesn't grasp their interest.

- May prefer 'big talk' to 'small talk'.

- May see interactions as a way to convey and receive information.

- May have difficulty with sarcasm, innuendo or other subtleties of language/interaction.

- May, or may have as a child, felt they were the 'last one to get the joke'.

- May have a low social battery that needs a lot more time to recharge.

- May find that people say their facial expressions do not match their emotional state.

- May have difficulty smiling for photos on demand.

- May find praise makes them uncomfortable.

- May find presents/surprises and similar forms of attention cause them discomfort.

- May have difficulty with hugs, handshakes, etc.

- May need to look away to think, process or form a response.

- May have difficulty modulating the rate, rhythm, tone or volume of their voice.

- May tend to adopt the phrases, mannerisms or accents of others, even subconsciously.

Social imagination

- May need structure and routine.

- May become angry or distressed at unexpected changes.

- May need to plan in advance (sometimes to the smallest detail!).

- May get anxious about going places even when they want to.

- May have difficulty instinctively knowing what others are thinking and feeling.

- May find they can be taken advantage of.

- May find they don't always realise the consequences of actions, which can be dangerous.

- May have difficulty with the 'unwritten' rules in the world.

Sensory differences

- May have difficulty recognising when hungry, thirsty or full.

- May find clothing irritating (may buy lots of same items when they find something tolerable).

- May experience sensitivity to noise.

- May love being in water – or avoid it!

- May have difficulty focusing on one thing – and/or be distracted by small sounds/movements.

- May have difficulty regulating their own temperature.

- May need time to process what has been said.

- May be sensitive to light.

- May be tactile seeking – for instance, like lots of fluffy blankets or different texture cushions that they can touch and weigh themselves down with.

- May always have the subtitles on the TV or need to write things down to process them.

- May have aversions to food textures and flavours.

- May find they cannot wear perfume, or use scented soaps or flavoured toothpastes.

Executive function, central coherence

- May have difficulty completing everyday tasks.

- Might often be late or miss appointments.

- May struggle to know where to start tasks.

- May be good at compartmentalising.

- May forget what they are doing or why they came into a room.

- May start lots of projects/crafts/hobbies they get very involved in and never finish…

- May lose belongings frequently.

- May experience daily living difficulties such as when preparing food – burning things, melting things, leaving things out of the fridge.

Emotional regulation

- May be extremely sensitive to the emotions of others – hyper empathetic.

- May be prone to frequent and dramatic mood shifts.

- May be prone to anxious thoughts or depressive states.

- May experience extreme excitement at seemingly small things.

- May experience significant sensitivity to rejection.

- May be unpredictable at times.

Other factors

Whilst supporting undiagnosed, suspected autistic people, it is important to bear in mind that autistic adults may have a history of:

- difficulties in education

- struggling to obtain or maintain appropriate employment that ensures they reach their full potential

- missing or being late for social engagements, appointments, etc.

- difficulties in maintaining self-care (e.g. keeping up with personal hygiene/grooming, shopping, cooking)

- difficulties around the home, in completing chores such as cleaning

- struggling to keep their environment and belongings organised

- difficulties making decisions

- find travel hard, such as utilising public transport or driving

- strengths and needs that are mismatched (a spiky profile).

Although we do not know the exact cause of autism, it is clear that there is a strong genetic component. This can mean that having family members who are autistic can be one indicator (in conjunction with other signs) that assessment is warranted.

Everyone will identify with some characteristics – autistic behaviours are human behaviours calibrated differently. This doesn't mean everyone is 'a little bit autistic' – the characteristics must meet a certain level, be pervasive and impact functioning.

If you are reading this book as an individual who is exploring the idea of an autism assessment for yourself, we have provided some useful tips and advice.

Pre-diagnosis – how can someone seeking assessment prepare?

- Read lots of autistic people's accounts, blogs, books, articles (there are some great books by non-autistic people too which can supplement this).

- Make lists with examples – gather evidence, including childhood history, school reports, developmental milestones, etc.

- Ask others for input (parents, partners, friends).

Making the referral

This differs in different countries. You can now self-refer to the Integrated Autism Services in Wales as an adult. While there is no unifying body or overarching network in the other UK nations, the National Autistic Society or Autistic Self Advocacy Network (https://autisticadvocacy.org) or Autistic Minds (Autistic Directory) could provide area-specific advice for seeking a diagnosis.

People with complex profiles/coexisting conditions may be assessed by or in conjunction with other professionals/services such as mental health services.

During diagnosis – what will happen and how?

Once you have made your referral, you will be screened and either placed on to the waiting list for consultation and assessment or contacted for further information, discussion or referral to other appropriate services.

Waiting time

Unfortunately, the time you wait for assessment and diagnosis can be extensive.

This can be difficult emotionally and can increase anxiety. You can ask the provider for your position on the list and the likely estimated wait time.

Diagnostic assessment

When you reach the top of the waiting list, you will receive an appointment for assessment and possible diagnosis.

The diagnostic tool used will depend on a range of factors, including the clinician's judgement, the method used by the team conducting the assessment, your age, complexity of profile and other factors. Sometimes more than one diagnostic tool will be used in collecting and assessing information. Commonly used tools include:

- DISCO: Diagnostic Interview for Social and Communication Disorders

- ADOS: Autism Diagnostic Observation Schedule

- ADIR: Autism Diagnostic Interview – Revised.

All of this can be very emotional and draining, and you may experience a range of feelings.

The assessment itself can take hours, it can involve recounting lots of memories and challenges, and hearing others describe things you struggle with.

You may not get an answer immediately. You may get your diagnosis at the assessment; alternatively,you may come back for a follow-up appointment, or receive information in the post.

It may be that the professionals feel you need further assessment or that your profile needs to be discussed/assessed by a multidisciplinary team/panel which may include:

- psychiatrist/psychologist

- occupational therapist (OT)

- speech and language therapist (SALT)

- other specialist professionals/trained diagnosticians.

Second opinions

Clinical experience, the diagnostic tools used and many other factors can impact the likelihood of you obtaining a diagnosis.

This can be disheartening, and some people may feel the diagnosis (or lack of) is not correct.

It can be good to take time to process what you have been told. If you are still sure you want to proceed with aiming to obtain a (different) diagnosis, you might decide to request a second opinion, or for more detailed information as to why you did not meet the criteria for diagnosis.

Post-diagnosis: coping with feelings and disclosing diagnosis

You may experience many different emotions during and post-diagnosis – ranging from happiness and relief to grief, confusion and/or anger. There is no one right way to feel or process the diagnosis. So be kind to yourself and allow yourself time and space to work through your emotions, whatever they may be. You are essentially reprocessing your life up to this point through a new lens, with the perspective of new information, or what I call a 'Tale of Two Yous' – the 'you' you thought you were, versus the 'you' you are beginning to understand. This can all be a real roller coaster of lightbulb moments and self-discovery.

Dealing with disclosure: key things to consider

Gill Loomes once wrote about 'kitchen sink moments'. That is, it's not only the big, one-off revelations where you reveal your diagnosis, but also the small moments, where you have to decide whether disclosure is safe, needed or wanted in that moment. Both types of disclosure can be tricky, and for some people, they may be safer and more comfortable than for others. Key things to consider may include:

- Do I want them to know?

- Do I need them to know?

- How might they react?

- How will I cope with their reaction?

If you decide to disclose, it can be helpful to give it thought beforehand – who am I telling, when am I telling them? – thinking through and preparing what to say as well as planning for their potential responses and how you will cope with the aftermath of disclosure.

Moving forward

Consider the following when moving forward post-diagnosis:

- Embracing the benefits of understanding yourself and finding your place in the autistic community.

- What help is out there for autistic adults?

  - Social care: Check out your local authority website for services available to you or reach out to an advocate who can help you access them.

  - Reasonable adjustments: These are a legal right in work and healthcare – research from trusted sources such as the Maternity and Autism Research Group, Birthrights or your local maternity professionals can help you plan and demand reasonable adjustments.

– Post-diagnostic counselling: These differ by local area so if you are not provided with post-diagnostic counselling after your assessment, contact your diagnosing professional for further advice.

– Financial assistance: Whether this is for a personal assistant, adaptations at home or at work can be helped with full or partial funding – contact your local authority or employer for more information. There are specific welfare benefits available for neurodivergent or disabled people whose condition impacts their ability to carry out daily care tasks. Welfare rights advisors or the Citizens Advice Bureau may be able to offer guidance and support with these matters, and there are useful websites which explain various benefits and entitlements such as TurntoUs or EntitledTo.

Keep learning! Take your voyage of discovery through learning about autism and other autistic people's experiences.

Apply this to your life, your history, your current strengths and difficulties, and use it for your future happiness!

Self-diagnosis or self-identifying

Some people are happy to research independently and engage with other autistic people to feel secure in self-diagnosis. This can have the benefit of not facing barriers to diagnosis and the logistical, emotional and sometimes financial challenges the process can present. They can still use this information to learn about and understand themselves, their lives, strengths, challenges and needs, and find and/or develop coping strategies accordingly.

Formal diagnosis

Others may feel they need the confirmation of the assessment and official diagnosis. For some people, this can be useful in obtaining support, and some people find that the process itself can be cathartic and reassuring.

Some 'top tips' for maternity/healthcare professionals

- Dim harsh lighting.

- Avoid strong smells where possible.

- Tour birthing site beforehand – familiarisation visits.

- Provide a 'photo map' of staff with names and job titles to help reduce anxiety.

- Knock before entering the room.

- Reduce language and allow processing time.

- Offer a choice of communication methods, such as visual aids.

- Offer positive sensory input, such as fidget toys.

- Recommend patient brings some favourite items for comfort.

- Offer soft music or meditation tracks.

- Keep the number of people (staff) in the room as low as possible.

- Consult with the carer/partner/family member where possible.

- Ask permission before touching or examining the patient *every* time.

- Clearly explain what is happening and why, and where possible what is likely to happen next.

- Be patient when answering questions.

- Be respectful and ensure the patient is involved in decisions about their care.

- Consider completing a patient profile in consultation with the patient and anyone present from their support network.

- Try to maintain continuity of staff where possible.

- Remember that pain may present differently and do not be dismissive.

- Encourage the patient to complete a birthing plan and, wherever possible, stick to it.

- Be mindful that there may be past trauma and/or heightened sensitivity to touch when conducting examinations.

- Where possible, provide information and resources for the patient to look at and process – then allow time for questions if needed.

- Consider the use of an autism-specific 'toolkit' (Nicolaidis *et al.* 2016).

- It is important to remember that adaptations may be necessary in the postnatal period also. Breastfeeding, for example, may pose specific sensory challenges for those with sensory sensitivity.

- Avoid metaphors – remember to keep language clear with as little room for misinterpretation as possible.

- Silence equipment where possible.

Autistic advocacy: accessible rights during pregnancy and motherhood

It is vital for all birthing people to be aware of their rights during pregnancy and childbirth but, as we have explored throughout the book, it may be of even more importance for those who are disabled and/or neurodivergent as unfortunately for many reasons our rights may not always be upheld and our needs may not always be met. This section aims to give easily understandable information about what your key rights are, how to access further information and how to assert your rights and/or seek support or further action if and when necessary. Some of this information will change over time, but the key agencies listed and underpinning legislation, guidance and case law should remain relevant. We are not legal professionals but we hope that this information serves as a starting point to help you feel more empowered and confident in knowing your rights and advocating for yourself/your loved ones. (**Note:** Some health and care policies may be affected due to the Covid-19 pandemic – in this case, please ask your healthcare provider how and why these adjustments have been made and if they are necessary.)

The guidance and legislation that protects you during pregnancy, childbirth and throughout healthcare may change over time, but current laws and guidelines that are currently of specific relevance are not limited to but may include:

- Equality Act 2010 – more information available via:
  - www.equalityhumanrights.com/en/equality-act

- – www.gov.uk/guidance/equality-act-2010-guidance
- European Convention on Human Rights – more information available via:
  - – www.echr.coe.int/documents/d/echr/Convention_ENG
- (enshrined in UK Law as the) Human Rights Act 1998 – more information available via:
  - – www.equalityhumanrights.com/en/human-rights/human-rights-act
- Mental Capacity Act 2005 – more information available via:
  - – www.legislation.gov.uk/ukpga/2005/9/contents
- Convention on the Elimination of Discrimination Against Women (CEDAW) – more information available via:
  - – www.ohchr.org/en/treaty-bodies/cedaw
- NMC (Nursing and Midwifery Council) code – more information available via:
  - – www.nmc.org.uk/standards/code
- NICE (National Institute for Health and Care Excellence) guidance – more information available via:
  - – nice.org.uk
- NHS patient rights (guidance may vary among devolved nations, i.e. England, Wales, Scotland, Ireland, and different rules may apply for non-UK citizens) – more information available via:
  - – www.nhs.uk/using-the-nhs/about-the-nhs/your-choices-in-the-nhs
  - – www.gov.uk/government/publications/the-nhs-choice-framework/the-nhs-choice-framework-what-choices-are-available-to-me-in-the-nhs
  - – https://nwssp.nhs.wales/a-wp/governance-e-manual/living-public-service-values/equality-diversity-and-human-rights
  - – www.nhsinform.scot/care-support-and-rights/health-rights

- www.nidirect.gov.uk/articles/your-rights-health

There are various agencies that could provide advice and support, such as the Citizens Advice Bureau (www.citizensadvice.org.uk/health/get-ad-vice-about-health-services), or specific charities/agencies for mental health, disability, gender and sexuality, etc.

More information on your rights during pregnancy and childbirth can be found at Birthrights, the UK's leading charity on human rights in child-birth, at Birthrights.org.uk. Birthrights have a wide range of freely available resources including factsheets, which are available in a range of languages and updated periodically. They also offer an email advice service for those whose queries have not been covered by their existing resources.

Key rights during pregnancy and childbirth
The right to medical care

In the UK, healthcare is seen as a fundamental human right. We have a National Health Service (NHS), which often provides this care, though some people may opt to pay for privately available treatment and care. The NHS constitution for England states that it 'provides a comprehensive service, available to all, irrespective of gender, race, disability, age, sexual orien-tation, religion, belief, gender reassignment, pregnancy and maternity or marital or civil partnership status'.

The right to have your fundamental needs met

You always have the right to have your basic needs met, for example access to food, water, toileting facilities and adequate pain relief. If pain relief is not given, there should be a valid reason for withholding it. If you feel your needs are not being met, you can complain to the primary healthcare professional or service manager.

The right to make choices, have a voice in your own care and give or decline consent

Healthcare professionals should make every effort to present information about your health and care in a way you can understand, including making reasonable adjustments in how they do this where possible, for example adjusting their language/communication or supporting information with visuals. You have the right to be given full and clear information about your care at every step in the process to allow you to evaluate fully and make the right choices for you. You should not feel rushed or pressured or that your opinions or need for more information are unimportant.

Often in healthcare and maternity care we find ourselves defaulting to what is known as the 'language of permission'. For example, 'I was not allowed a home birth' or 'they did not let me choose a water birth'. Of even more concern, sometimes birthing people, particularly those with vulnerabilities, feel pressured into making choices against their wishes or feel they are unable to refuse treatment or specific courses of action. For example, you may have been 'strongly advised' against a particular course of action such as home birth where healthcare professionals have told you 'it is safer for you and the baby in a hospital'. Often this advice has clear basis in your overall health profile and risk factors, and any decision should be explored and weighed carefully with full input from your healthcare team, but you always have the right to give or decline consent, even against medical advice. This includes examinations, treatment and where and how you give birth. It is important to note that under UK law, a foetus does not have rights and a baby only becomes a separate entity with its own legal rights after birth, so you are able to make decisions about your body and cannot be forced to accept treatment or take a particular course of action based on the needs of your unborn child.

As a rule, maternity services should 'start from yes' in your choices about your care and always have a good reason if they feel they need to say no. Just as at any other time in your life, your body belongs to you and consent is key – no means no. The only time that medical professionals can override your wishes is if you are not able to make a decision. This could be because you are incapacitated or unconscious due to an emergency situation or, in rare cases, because you are unable to understand the choices and the potential consequences of a decision even after it is very clearly explained – this is where it can be decided you do not have mental capacity.

Mental capacity should be considered on a decision-by-decision basis and you should be supported to make your own decisions as far as possible. Being autistic, disabled or having a mental health condition does not automatically mean you lack capacity. There is clear guidance and frameworks for healthcare professionals to assess capacity and lack of capacity should never be assumed without clear evidence. In some cases, where it is found you lack capacity, someone else may make decisions about your care. This may be a healthcare professional or a loved one. In some cases a loved one may have what is known as a 'Lasting Power of Attorney', which enables them to make decisions about your health and welfare, or your property and financial affairs. Mental capacity is a complex topic and it should be noted the information given above applies to those over 18 years old, but more information on mental capacity can be found at:

- www.gov.uk/government/publications/mental-capacity-act-code-of-practice

- www.birthrights.org.uk/factsheets/mental-capacity-and-maternity-care

- www.nhs.uk/conditions/social-care-and-support-guide/making-decisions-for-someone-else/mental-capacity-act

The right to be treated with dignity and have your privacy respected

You have the right to feel respected at all times, which includes healthcare professionals treating you with politeness and respecting your views and beliefs. It also means healthcare professionals should endeavour to support you to make informed decisions about your care. This may include making reasonable adjustments to help you to do this. You also have the right to privacy, for example when breast/chestfeeding.

The right to complain

You have the right to complain if you do not feel your treatment met your needs and/or wishes.

There are Patient Liaison Services (PALS) that can help with your complaint. You may complain to the specific healthcare provider or service, the local health board or the NHS commissioner. In some cases where you do not feel this has resolved the issue you may complain to the relevant ombudsman, or in some cases you may feel the need to seek independent legal advice. More information on how to complain can be found at:

- www.nhs.uk/contact-us/give-feedback-or-make-complaint

- www.nhs.uk/nhs-services/hospitals/what-is-pals-patient-advice-and-liaison-service

- www.healthwatch.co.uk/your-local-healthwatch/list

- www.birthrights.org.uk/factsheets/making-a-complaint

- www.ombudsman.org.uk/making-complaint

CHAPTER 8

Summary and Closing Wishes

Our master's degrees have opened the door to a previously shrouded world of science and academia. The mere fact that training ourselves in this discipline has introduced us to knowledge, advocacy and more effective activism has reinforced our belief that research should be accessible and widely disseminated, and should have value for the lives of those it focuses on. It is our strong belief that we shouldn't have to be on this side of the 'podium' to be heard.

On a personal level, we as parents have become increasingly incensed at the treatment we received and the resulting effects during the birth of our children. We realise what a difference small adjustments, understanding and empathy would have made to us and our families, and this has only increased our determination to increase knowledge and resources in health-care in sexual health, pregnancy, birth, parenting and healthcare generally.

It has been truly cathartic to take an experience that made us feel weak, insignificant, afraid and disempowered, and work through it professionally and personally with a critical eye and a logical mind, and realise that we did not fail, but rather we were failed, as so many others have been and continue to be.

It is emboldening and encouraging to have our voices heard, finally, after years of 'screaming into the abyss', and to utilise our own experiences in the hope of helping others. It gives meaning to an otherwise avoidable trauma.

Our professional feedback and evaluations have combined to create a rebuff to all the negative messages, microaggressions and internalised ableism we have collected over the years, reassuring us that we are not worthless, lazy, fragile or a burden. We are just autistic and misunderstood.

It is clear that pregnancy, birth and new motherhood can be a stressful, emotional and trying time for any woman, and those around her. All women can face gender disparities in healthcare, a patriarchal attitude to their choices and ingrained, systemic issues around consent, reproductive rights and their importance beyond that of a 'vessel' designed to ensure the arrival of a healthy baby above all else.

When a woman is facing additional or multiple disadvantages, these challenges can be compounded, leading to ever more threats to autonomy, dignity, respect and their voice in their own person-centred care that seems to be a common thread in policy, guidance and, indeed, ethos, but that can be, in practice, difficult to achieve when faced by the barriers of stigma, lack of training, time and financial constraints, and an increasingly stressed system which has been shown to not only fail its patients, but also its professionals.

It seems that with the differences in neurotype that being autistic brings, there come additional, specific needs, and some may say strengths, but certainly a need for differentiated care in order to reach the best outcome for all.

Autistic women's social, sensory and processing differences need to be accounted for, understood and supported during a time of great change, transition and anxiety. When consideration is given to the likelihood of pre-existing mental health or other co-occurring conditions, prior trauma or a history of finding appropriate healthcare difficult to access, this is additionally imperative.

With this in mind, we need more research on autistic women's experiences of pregnancy, birth and motherhood, to broaden our knowledge, and, essentially, we need this to be truly co-produced, thus bringing the insight only participatory research can yield. After all, key to this topic remaining overlooked for so long is that autistic women were considered invisible, unheard, misunderstood.

We need a framework for healthcare that means essential needs are understood and met, that caring for autistic women, for those with mental health conditions, with prior trauma, who are coping with multiple disadvantage or the intersectionality of marginalisation of neurotype, disability, race, culture, sexuality, gender and language barriers is not an 'added extra' but fundamental to our ethos of quality, person-centred care.

We can build upon the precedent of perinatal mental health teams, of specialist midwives for substance abuse, domestic violence and ethnic minorities, and research that shows autistic people are at a disadvantage in health, care and mortality, whilst capitalising on the political momentum around autism and neurodiversity to demand better.

In a system where we face injured people waiting hours for ambulances and dying in hospital corridors, and the loss of seasoned professionals due to burnout every day, to some people, such accommodations may seem frivolous, icing on a cake we are barely able to bake. With consultants suggesting mandatory training has 'metastasised' throughout the health service like an aggressive cancer, will additional demands for training, resources and specialism be met with disdain, reluctance or exhaustion? The answer is maybe. In some cases, probably.

But we can only make change one step at a time, and for every professional who is engaged, who expands their knowledge, their empathy and their understanding, we provide the spark for an improved maternity care experience for many women.

The day you meet your child should be joyful, exuberant, empowering and, above all else, a cherished memory. We owe that to women, to their loved ones and to their ability to heal and bond with their babies. We owe it to the wider narrative about what is important, about dignity, respect, feminism and a culture of care that evolves from both triumphs and mistakes. Instead of a society which blanches at the thought of admitting mistakes and the need for improvements, we can promote true reflective practice, transparency and a commitment to continually enhancing our knowledge, sensitivity and ultimately the care we provide, the lives we impact.

We need to champion continuity of care, continued professional development, and we need avenues for professionals on the 'ground' to evaluate, monitor and effectively feed back what they see. We need to provide clear avenues of support, guidance and opportunities to share positive and negative experiences – particularly where women may find additional barriers in navigating bureaucracy or advocating for themselves.

We need training around autism and neurodiversity in healthcare as can be seen from the disparity in health, care and mortality. We need this training ideally to be high quality, current, robust and co-produced, with a framework for ensuring the content is up to par. In maternity care, this training has the potential to make a huge difference, to autistic women, and also to their partners and loved ones.

We need clear communication, pathways, environmental adjustments and quality resources – and this good practice can benefit everyone. What woman navigating maternity care would not benefit from clear information, visual reinforcement and resources that help her have a voice in her own care? These accommodations could be specifically beneficial for those with mental health conditions such as anxiety, those with intellectual disabilities, those for whom English is a second language…the possibilities are endless.

This work has been the result of highly personal trauma, which we have relived, wished away and been angered by. It is an intensely personal experience that was once needlessly traumatic, which left us feeling disempowered, ashamed, guilty, weak and robbed of what should have been in many ways beautiful. Throughout the course of our master's, our essays, our professional work, both training and speaking, we have remembered, relieved and rewritten every awful moment, sometimes in toe-curling, anxiety-inducing, high-definition detail. We have begun to accept what happened to us, and what has likely happened to so many others, and to find the beauty and usefulness in it. Our aim is to highlight these issues, to develop our work, to drive our activism and to ensure that, above all, our trauma has value, in reducing the likelihood of other women experiencing similar.

Regardless of impact, or any success in highlighting the issues, in encouraging further research or training, this reflection has given us immense personal growth, empowerment and the opportunity to start reclaiming some of what was lost to us. It is our dearest hope that it prevents other women from having to struggle as we did, that it opens a much-needed conversation that ultimately leads to positive change.

Emma's Birth Experience

My partner (P) and I had agreed to start a family around 18 months before I became pregnant. We had both experienced difficult childhoods, and therefore we embarked on the journey to become parents with the deep-rooted goal of doing it right.

I had a history of mental health and physical issues dating back to my pre-teen years. However, the only confirmed diagnoses I had then received were depression, anxiety and social phobia.

I coped with pregnancy adequately. There were visuals and descriptions available of what to expect week by week, clear rules to follow. I struggled slightly physically, and of course I was anxious, but even ceasing my anti-depressants did not seem to affect my mood too drastically.

I was terrified of childbirth, though – of being in a strange, bright, noisy, unpredictable environment. The prenatal classes echoed my research on caring for a newborn but didn't cover what to expect during labour in detail. I read women's accounts of labour, but they tended to be more descriptive of feelings than the actual process. As time passed, my anxiety increased, and I requested a home water birth. This request was denied, the midwives insisting hospital was safer. I asked my consultant about an elective caesarean, but he advised against this.

We agreed I would attend the midwife-led birth centre. It was local and familiar, and the staff allowed us to look around in advance. It was decorated more like a hotel than a hospital, and, most importantly, P would be allowed to stay throughout.

I made a birth plan, advising that P was to advocate for me if I was unable, pain relief would be as needed, and, most desirable of all, I wished to use the birthing pool.

I suffered severe pain in the days before labour, as the sciatica and pelvic pain present throughout my pregnancy intensified. Then at 3 am, I woke suddenly and my waters broke.

P rang the midwife, who advised us to stay home as long as possible, to rest if we could. We were told baths were unadvisable, as there was a risk of infection as my waters had broken. They said to attend at 8 am for an examination.

When we attended, I gave the midwives my list of contractions. They were fluctuating between strong, long contractions and short, weak and intermittent. The midwives seemed dubious of this information, and of my self-reported pain levels, suggesting this was 'unlikely' as I was only 2cm dilated. They advised I go home and relax, stating that they 'did not want to see me before 12 noon'.

By 11.30 am I couldn't stand the pain, curled up in agony, sure I must have progressed. We returned to the birth centre. Upon arrival, the midwife chastised me, 'I said I didn't want to see you before 12!'

I explained I was finding the pain unbearable, but the midwife replied they could not administer pain relief until I was 4cm dilated. I requested she check; she replied she would if I insisted, but 'repeated examinations were a bad idea'. She found I hadn't progressed much and said there was nothing they could do at present. She said, 'Well, since you've made me examine you, I will give you a sweep, maybe that will move things along.' The sweep hurt, and I squirmed backwards up the bed. She said tersely that she knew it was uncomfortable, but I needed to deal with it. She asked me to go home, or for a walk along the beach. I refused. I was in a lot of pain, distressed, even more uncomfortable in public than usual. I tried to walk around the hospital's top floor, near the birth unit, but was desperate to get back to our quiet room there, away from people.

The staff made it clear they were unhappy I wanted to stay, saying I was making it harder on myself by not going home. Several staff came in and out of the room, admonishing me for being there, with comments like 'I bet you didn't even try to have a bath' despite my being advised against this. I was told the birthing pool wasn't an option.

Once the staff realised I was determined to stay, they left the room. I was very agitated at this point, uncomfortable in this environment but more terrified still of being home with no medical assistance. My pain and distress were reaching unbearable levels, but rather than inspiring sympathy and compassion, this seemed to annoy and frustrate the staff. I was told that if I wasn't coping now, I would never cope later.

Eventually, a different midwife entered. Seeing I was very upset, she tried to calm me. She suggested a bath would be OK and prepared one in the adjoining bathroom. This helped a little, but only for a short time. This midwife then said her shift was ending.

I paced the room, panicking and panting, unable to control my anxiety. I was in agony. P asked the midwife for help, but she said she could do nothing. I asked for a TENS machine at least; sighing, she said it was a nuisance, but she would see what she could find. She came back a while later saying she had managed to get one.

The TENS machine helped slightly at first, but was soon at maximum, yet I could barely feel it through the pain. I was hysterical now, P pleading with me to calm down, afraid for both me and the baby. He called the midwife again and I begged her for pain relief. She said, 'Well, the baby's facing the wrong way to start with. Have you even tried crouching on all fours?' Crying, I replied no one had stated this before, so no. Exasperated, she told me to try it and she would return shortly.

She returned with a needle, saying she had 'a little something to calm you down'. I asked what it was and she reiterated 'something to calm you'. I asked again. She replied that it was a half dose of pethidine. I asked if it could be administered if I wasn't 4cm, but she said it was OK, so I agreed.

The pethidine made me drowsy, and P helped me into bed. I drifted briefly but soon awoke abruptly. Rushing to the bathroom, I suddenly needed to push. I heard a loud, strange, noise and I realised, shocked, it was coming from me.

Midwives flooded in and helped me to the bed, seeming shocked at this sudden progression. I couldn't stop screaming. One midwife looked me straight in the eye, saying, 'Scream all you want, you will only lose your voice.'

They gave me gas and air. This helped slightly, though I kept biting the nozzle off in panic. The midwives said I wasn't coping, suggesting we travel to Bridgend Hospital where they could administer an epidural. I agreed.

The ambulance arrived, and the paramedic was kind. He held my hand, advising me to breathe slowly and deeply so the gas and air would work better. I did. Once at the ambulance, we were told P couldn't travel with us, as there wasn't room with the paramedic and midwife. P followed by car.

In the ambulance, my contractions were subsiding, and I could speak at times. The midwife seemed nervous, telling me not to push. I heard her ask the paramedic if there was a birth kit on board; he said no. I panicked because P wasn't here. I asked if the baby was coming. She said no, but still seemed nervous, tutting when we slowed in traffic. The lights and sirens were on now.

Suddenly, we were at the hospital, and I was swinging my head around wildly, looking for P. The midwife was tapping the elevator button frantically, muttering. Then, as the doors opened, P appeared.

We were soon in a delivery room. I requested an epidural but it was too late. New midwives joined us and everything happened fast. My daughter emerged, the cord briefly wrapped around her neck, before the midwife swiftly untangled her.

She was placed on my chest. I looked at her. Everything was surreal. I asked P to hold her while I was stitched. The midwife from Port Talbot was leaving and I remember apologising profusely for being so difficult. I can't remember her reply.

A student midwife helped me to the bathroom. She was kind, careful. She offered to help me shower, getting permission to assist me each step of the way.

The staff agreed we could return to Port Talbot for postnatal care, as I was agitated at the thought of P having to leave.

Another midwife was at the birth centre when we returned. She said the baby needed to feed and, without asking, removed my top. She began squeezing, saying she needed to coax my milk supply.

In the following days, my distress continued. I felt detached, confused, lost. Staff came into the room without knocking. I begged to go home but was persuaded to stay for three days.

We went home but I continued to struggle. P was unable to leave me alone, and small tasks like attempting to use the steriliser were enough to cause hysterics. I had to be reminded to eat each spoon of my food. My daughter seemed to scream constantly, feeding was problematic, and I was terrified of hurting her when handling her.

A visiting midwife suggested I had post-traumatic stress disorder (PTSD). P was unable to work until our daughter was nine months old, then only on a part-time basis. The effects were substantial and lasting.

It is hard to describe the sheer terror and panic I felt during childbirth. I blamed myself for a long time for not being good enough, strong enough, for putting such pressure on P, for failing.

I had perceived the midwives as hostile, cruel, feeling they hated me, yet blaming myself for invoking their reactions with my weakness.

I had been desperate to escape the birth environment, sure that if I could only go home, the world would make sense again, but it didn't. My home was gone, a new, distorted version in its place. Although our baby fascinated me, evoking overwhelming feelings of protectiveness and love, I was unable to adjust to this tiny stranger inserted into our lives. I alternated between catatonia and hysterics for weeks. I relived my screams during childbirth every time my daughter cried, which was often. I felt violated, ravaged, physically and emotionally.

I seemed to lack the maternal instinct that society tells us women are meant to have. I felt guilt, shame, despair, and fell completely to pieces, unable to regulate my emotions or master my pain. I was completely dependent on P, mortified at his far superior parenting instincts.

Evaluating this experience, analysing these feelings in the context of my late ASD diagnosis, and my increasing understanding of autism, I can finally begin to forgive myself this huge list of inadequacies. I can understand the differences in functioning that led to such difficulty adjusting, processing, regulating. Reading my account as impartially as is possible, I can feel sympathy for the struggles I faced, and disappointment and frustration at a maternity system that contributed to rather than lessened these struggles.

I look back now at the confused, scared version of myself that lived this experience, and I realise that sharing this condition, a condition that can be both a burden and a privilege, has ignited a fire inside me. I feel a sense of injustice, for this past version of myself and for other autistic women, particularly those who may not have been blessed with support, and the opportunity to educate and therefore empower themselves as I have. It sounds like a cliché but it is truly genuine to say that I now feel that in some way each battle I fight for myself may make the battle in some way easier for who comes next, and that feeling makes me stronger, more determined. I now understand that I was not mad, bad, or useless, but coping with a difference as deep as my neurology. Having begun to learn my rights, and how to apply them, I will never allow myself to be so disempowered again. I feel a thread of invisible support from all these other women, struggling just as I have, and in that recognition, there is relief and belonging at last.

A partner's role

For me, the presence of my partner felt as necessary as oxygen. I'm not using dramatic licence when I say that; he provides me with a sense of safety, a buffer to the outside world that is often extremely difficult, distressing and sometimes downright impossible to navigate. I withdraw when I 'reach my limit', which happens for me much sooner than it does for someone without autism or mental health conditions, and is triggered by seemingly nonsensical things that I often don't comprehend myself.

The thought of being in the birth environment alone, without him, was so unimaginably awful to me. This was a huge factor in choosing the midwife-led birth centre for labour and delivery, as he could stay with us throughout the process, and in the days afterwards, which we were told he would not have been able to do at the hospital maternity wards. I should state that I find unpredictable interactions with people I do not know disconcerting and nerve-wracking under the most innocuous circumstances, such as a meter reader knocking on my door, or a neighbour calling to me for some reason as a I walk to my car. Yet here I was faced with what seemed like an endless stream of unknown faces, voices and personalities completely foreign to me, all in one of the most vulnerable situations you can think of.

I remember at points during labour being in a strange state, alternating between hazily catching information from the environment and people around me and listening to the sounds of my own guttural screams, a noise I had not even known I could make until that day. The sound and sensation was terrifying to me, and yet I could not stop. At several points in my active labour, I was rendered completely unable to communicate, left completely dependent on my partner to be my voice in this environment which I perceived as hostile, confusing and overwhelming.

The pressure he must have felt, the helplessness and the immense responsibility fills me with both guilt and gratitude and love. Although rationally there was never a threat to my life, I can honestly say I felt that threat on a primitive level. I could not reason myself out of it. There were points where I was so overwhelmed and afraid that I wished for death, a thought that now fills me with horror, dread and shame, for in so casually wishing for the end of my existence, I gave no thought to the life I was entrusted to protect, the life that grew into the beautiful daughter I cherish above all else.

A partner's perspective

As my research strongly suggested that the impact the birth experience had on me, my partner (P) and our relationship was shared by others, particularly the rippling impact on partners, I felt it important to ask him about his feelings and recollections of the event, and include a summary here.

P said that he found his recall of the specifics of our daughter's birth and first few weeks postpartum hazy at first, although key themes were immediately accessible.

P remembered, primarily, feeling responsible for the emotional and physical wellbeing of me and our daughter. He said that he didn't really have time to overthink what was happening, so focused was he on this responsibility. Indeed, during early labour he was genuinely fearful for the impact my increasingly agitated state was having on me and our baby.

He recalled feeling pushed aside, ignored, like a 'non-entity', by the birthing team. He felt frustration at the attitude towards us, which was, at best, indifferent and even, at times, hostile.

He said that it was incredibly difficult to watch someone you love going through such pain and distress, whilst feeling so helpless yourself.

P perceived a lack of respect for our privacy during childbirth and in the days that we spent at the birth centre afterwards. He found this frustrating and difficult to handle.

He felt that as a father he was not given any consideration at all during childbirth, an attitude that he feels has often persisted in the decade since our daughter's birth, despite him playing an active and integral role in our daughter's upbringing. This he finds insulting and frustrating, as he feel it minimises the valuable and equal contribution he has made to parenting our daughter.

He felt unable to ever face the traumatic experience of childbirth again, witnessing the pain and distress of a loved one, so much so that he requested his doctor refer him for a vasectomy less than a week after our daughter's birth. Although my efforts and those of the doctor persuaded him against such drastic action, time has proved that his initial resolution was not a rash decision.

Abbreviations

AAC	alternative/augmentative communication
ABA	applied behaviour analysis
ADHD	attention deficit hyperactivity disorder
APA	American Psychiatric Association
ARFID	avoidant/restrictive food intake disorder
ASD	autism spectrum disorder, broadly referred to throughout as autism
EDA/PDA	extreme or pathological demand avoidance, also sometimes referred to as 'demand-avoidant profiles'
EDS	Ehlers–Danlos syndrome
FII	fabricated or induced illness
HJS	hypermobility joint syndrome
HSD	hypermobility spectrum disorder
LD/ID	learning/intellectual disability
NHS	National Health Service
NMC	Nursing and Midwifery Council
OCD	obsessive compulsive disorder
ODD	oppositional defiant disorder
OT	occupational therapy/therapist
PBM	Positive Birth Movement
PDG	protodeclarative gestures
PTSD/CPTSD	post-traumatic stress disorder/complex post-traumatic stress disorder
PTSD-PC	post-traumatic stress disorder – post childbirth
RSD	rejection sensitivity dysphoria
SALT	speech and language therapy/therapist
SPD	symphysis pubis dysfunction
WHO	World Health Organization

References

AASPIRE (2023). AASPIRE Healthcare Toolkit. https://autismandhealth.org.

Abraham, E., Hendler, T., Zagoory-Sharon, O. & Feldman, R. (2019). Interoception sensitivity in the parental brain during the first months of parenting modulates children's somatic symptoms six years later: The role of oxytocin. *International Journal of Psychophysiology 136*, 39–48. doi:10.1016/j.ijpsycho.2018.02.001.

Adhiyaman, M. (2019). Mandatory training – the elephant in the room. *British Medical Journal Opinion*. https://blogs.bmj.com/bmj/2019/05/03/murthy-adhiyaman-mandatory-training-the-elephant-in-the-room.

Allely, C.S. (2013). Pain sensitivity and observer perception of pain in individuals with autism spectrum disorder. *Scientific World Journal 2013*, 916178. doi:10.1155/2013/916178.

Alston, P. (2018). OHCHR Statement on Visit to the United Kingdom, by Professor Philip Alston, United Nations Special Rapporteur on extreme poverty and human rights. www.ohchr.org/EN/NewsEvents/Pages/DisplayNews.aspx?NewsID=23881&LangID=E.

American Psychiatric Association (2013). *Diagnostic and Statistical Manual of Mental Disorders (DSM-5®)*. Arlington, VA: APA.

Andersson, D. (2021). New study shows Fibromyalgia likely the result of autoimmune problems. King's College London. www.kcl.ac.uk/news/new-study-shows-fibromyalgia-likely-the-result-of-autoimmune-problems.

Arnstein, S. (1969). A ladder of citizen participation. *Journal of the American Planning Association 35*(4), 216–224.

Appignanesi, L. (2008). *Mad, Bad and Sad: A History of Women and the Mind Doctors from 1800 to Present.* London: Virago Press.

Arnold, C. (2016). The invisible link between autism and anorexia. *Spectrum News*, 17 February. www.spectrumnews.org/features/deep-dive/the-invisible-link-between-autism-and-anorexia.

ASAN (2009). Why Autism Speaks does not speak for us. https://asancentralohio.blogspot.com/2009/08/why-autism-speaks-does-not-speak-for-us.html.

Autistic Empire (2023). Klein Sexual Orientation Grid. www.autisticempire.com/klein.

Autistic People Speaking Out (2013). Autistic and pregnant. https://autistics-speaking.tumblr.com/post/55965301552/autistic-and-pregnant.

Autistica (2016). Personal Tragedies, Public Crisis: The Urgent Need for a National Response to Early Death in Autism. www.autistica.org.uk/downloads/files/Personal-tragedies-public-crisis-ONLINE.pdf.

Autism West Midlands (2020). Food, Diet and Autism. www.autismwestmid-lands.org.uk/wp-content/uploads/2020/02/Food_Diet_and_Autism_Febru-ary_2020.pdf.

Autside Education and Training (2023). Use of language. https://autsideeducation.co.uk/use-of-language.

Baeza-Velasco, C., Cohen, D., Hamonet, C., Vlamynck, E. *et al.* (2018). Autism, joint hypermobility-related disorders and pain. *Frontiers in Psychiatry 9*. doi:10.3389/fpsyt.2018.00656.

Ballantyne, A. & Rogers, W. (2016). Pregnancy, Vulnerability, and the Risk of Exploitation in Clinical Research. In F. Baylis & A. Ballantyne (eds) *Clinical Research Involving Pregnant Women* (pp.139–159). Cham: Springer.

Bamber, J. (2003). Childbirth pain relief study reveals inequalities for BAME mothers. NHS 75, 9 March. www.cuh.nhs.uk/news/childbirth-pain-relief-study-reveals-inequalities-for-bame-mothers.

Bargiela, S., Steward, R. & Mandy, W. (2016). The experiences of late-diagnosed women with autism spectrum conditions: An investigation of the female autism phenotype. *Journal of Autism and Developmental Disorders 46*(10), 3281–3294. doi:10.1007/s10803-016-2872-8.

Baron-Cohen, S. (1989). The autistic child's theory of mind: A case of specific developmental delay. *Child Psychology & Psychiatry & Allied Disciplines 30*(2), 285–297.

Baron-Cohen, S. (2002). The extreme male brain theory of autism. *Trends in Cognitive Sciences 6*(6), 248–254. https://doi.org/10.1016/s1364-6613(02)01904-6.

Baron-Cohen, S. (2003). *The Essential Difference: Male and Female Brains and the Truth about Autism.* New York, NY: Basic Books.

Baron-Cohen, S. (2006). Empathy: Freudian origins and twenty-first century neuroscience. *Psychology 9*(19), 536–537.

Baron-Cohen, S. (2009). Autism: The empathizing-systemising (E-S) theory. *Annals of the New York Academy of Sciences 1156*, 68–80. doi:10.1111/j.1749-6632.2009.04467.x.

Baron-Cohen, S., Leslie, A.M. & Frith, U. (1985). Does the autistic child have 'Theory of Mind'? *Cognition 21*(1), 37–46. doi:10.1016/0010-0277(85)90022-8.

Bates, K., Goodley, D. & Runswick-Cole, K. (2017). Precarious lives and resistant possibilities: The labour of people with learning disabilities in times of austerity. *Disability & Society 32*(2), 160–175. doi:10.1080/09687599.2017.1281105.

BBC News (2019a). Judges overturn 'forced abortion' ruling. London, 24 June. www.bbc.co.uk/news/uk-england-london-48751067.

BBC News (2019b). New review into autistic teen's death. Bristol, 7 August. www.bbc.co.uk/news/uk-england-bristol-49250377.

Beardon, L. (2018). Three golden rules for supporting autistic pupils. *TES Magazine*, 7 November. www.tes.com/news/three-golden-rules-supporting-autistic-pupils.

Beebe, L. & Gossler, S. (2013). Nursing of autism spectrum disorder: Evidence-based integrated care across the lifespan. *Issues in Mental Health Nursing 34*(8), 631. doi:10.3109/01612840.2012.708706.

Begeer, S., El Bouk, S., Boussaid, W., Meerum Terwogt, M. & Koot, H.M. (2009). Underdiagnosis and referral bias of autism in ethnic minorities. *Journal of Autism and Developmental Disorders 39*(1), 142–148. doi:10.1007/s10803-008-0611-5.

Beggiato, A., Peyre, H., Maruani, A., Scheid, I. *et al.* (2017). Gender differences in autism spectrum disorders: Divergence among specific core symptoms. *Autism Research 10*(4), 680–689. doi:10.1002/aur.1715.

Belger, A., Carpenter, K.L.H. & Schipul, S.E. (2014). Imaging the Neural Correlates of Behavioral and Cognitive Shifts in Autism. In: Patel, V., Preedy, V., Martin, C. (eds) *Comprehensive Guide to Autism.* New York, NY: Springer.

Bennett, L. & Humphries, R. (2014). *Making Best Use of the Better Care Fund: Spending to Save?* The King's Fund. www.kingsfund.org.uk/sites/default/files/field/field_publication_file/making-best-use-of-the-better-care-fund-kingsfund-jan14.pdf.

Bever, L. (2019). How a 'Sesame Street' Muppet became embroiled in a controversy over autism. *Washington Post*, 19 September. www.washingtonpost.com/health/2019/09/19/how-sesame-street-muppet-became-embroiled-controversy-over-autism.

Birthrights (2013). *Dignity in Childbirth: Projects and Perspectives.* www.birthrights.org.uk/wp-content/uploads/2019/07/Birthrights-Projects-and-Perspectives.pdf.

Birthrights (2016). Disabled women and birthing people's experiences of maternity care. www.birthrights.org.uk/campaigns-research/disability.

Bishop-Fitzpatrick, L. & Kind, A.J.H. (2017). A scoping review of health disparities in autism spectrum disorder. *Journal of Autism and Developmental Disorders 47*, 3380–3391.

Bloom, A. (2008). *Closing of the American Mind.* New York, NY: Simon & Schuster.

Bloom, B. (1956). *Taxonomy of Educational Objectives: The Classification of Educational Goals.* New York, NY: David McKay.

Boal, A. (1993). Theatre of the Oppressed. In F. Babbage (ed.) *Augusto Boal* (pp.35–66). London: Routledge.

Botha, M. & Frost, D.M. (2020). Extending the minority stress model to understand mental health problems experienced by the autistic population. *Society and Mental Health 10*(1), 20–34. doi:10.1177/2156869318804297.

Boyer, K. (2018). *Spaces and Politics of Motherhood.* London: Rowman & Littlefield International.

Bradfield, Z., Hauck, Y., Duggan, R. & Kelly, M. (2019). Midwives' perceptions of being 'with woman': A phenomenological study. *BMC Pregnancy Childbirth 19*, 363. doi:10.1186/s12884-019-2548-4.

Bradley, R. & Slade, P. (2011). A review of mental health problems in fathers following the birth of a child. *Journal of Reproductive and Infant Psychology 29*(1), 19–42. doi:10.1080/02646838.2010.513047.

Bravo, J.F. & Wolff, C. (2006). Clinical study of hereditary disorders of connective tissues in a Chilean population. *Arthritis & Rheumatism 54*(2), 515–523.

Brigante, L. (2022). How birthplace and outcomes are evolving in England and Wales. Royal College of Midwives. www.rcm.org.uk/news-views/rcm-opinion/2022/how-birthplace-and-outcomes-are-evolving-in-england-wales.

Brouwer, M.E., Williams, A.D., Van Grinsven, S.E., Cuijpers, P. *et al.* (2018). Offspring outcomes after prenatal interventions for common mental disorders: A meta-analysis. *BMC Medicine 16*(1). doi:10.1186/s12916-018-1192-6.

Brown, A. (2021). *Breastfeeding Uncovered: Who Really Decides How We Feed Our Babies*, 2nd edn. London: Pinter & Martin.

Brown-Lavoie, S.M., Viecili, M.A. & Weiss, J.A. (2014). Sexual knowledge and victimization in adults with autism spectrum disorders. *Journal of Autism and Developmental Disorders 44*(9), 2185–2196. doi:10.1007/s10803-014-2093-y.

Buckley-Thomson, L. (2012). Court bans autistic woman from having sex. UK Human Rights Blog, 14 February. https://ukhumanrightsblog.com/2012/02/14/court-bans-autistic-woman-from-having-sex.

Burch, L. (2017). 'You are a parasite on the productive classes': Online disablist hate speech in austere times. *Disability & Society 33*(3), 392–415. doi:10.1080/09687599.2017.1411250.

Burstow, B. (2019). Autistic and Mad: Dialogue with Nick Walker. In B. Burstow (ed.) *The Revolt against Psychiatry: A Counterhegemonic Dialogue*. London: Palgrave Macmillan.

Burton, T. (2016). *Exploring the Experiences of Pregnancy, Birth and Parenting of Mothers with Autism Spectrum Disorder.* Doctoral thesis, Staffordshire University.

Butler, P. (2017). UK austerity policies 'amount to violations of disabled people's rights'. *The Guardian*, 28 November. www.theguardian.com/business/2016/nov/07/uk-austerity-policies-amount-to-violations-of-disabled-peoples-rights.

Byers, E.S., Nichols, S. & Voyer, S.D. (2013). Challenging stereotypes: Sexual functioning of single adults with high functioning autism spectrum disorder. *Journal of Autism and Developmental Disorders 43*(11), 2617–2627. doi:10.1007/s10803-013-1813-z.

Byrom, S. & Downe, S. (2015). *The Roar Behind the Silence: Why Kindness, Compassion and Respect Matter in Maternity Care*. London: Pinter & Martin.

Caldwell, L. & Grobbel, C.C. (2013). The importance of reflective practice in nursing. *International Journal of Caring Sciences 6*(3), 319–326.

Camaioni, L., Perucchini, P., Muratori, F., Parrini, B. & Cesari, A. (2003). The communicative use of pointing in autism: Developmental profile and factors related to change. *European Psychiatry 18*(1), 6–12.

Campbell, D., Duncan, P. & Marsh, S. (2018). NHS patients dying in hospital corridors, A&E doctors tell Theresa May. *The Guardian*, 11 January. www.theguardian.com/society/2018/jan/11/nhs-patients-dying-in-hospital-corridors-doctors-tell-theresa-may.

Campbell, M.A. (2020). *'This Distressing Malady': Childbirth and Mental Illness in Scotland 1820–1930*. PhD thesis, University of St Andrews. https://research-repository.st-andrews.ac.uk/handle/10023/19534.

Campbell, R. and Macfarlane, A. (1994). *Where To Be Born*. Oxford: National Perinatal Epidemiology Unit.

Carers UK (2014). *State of Caring 2014*. London: Carers UK. https://hscbusiness.hscni.net/pdf/State_of_caring_2014.pdf.

Carper, B.A. (1978). Fundamental patterns of knowing in nursing. *Advances in Nursing Science 1*(1), 13–24. doi:10.1097/00012272-197810000-00004.

Carter, J. & Duriez, T. (1986). *With Child: Birth through the ages*. Edinburgh: Mainstream Publishing Company.

Casanova, E.L., Baeza-Velasco, C., Buchanan, C.B. & Casanova, M.F. (2020). The relationship between autism and Ehlers-Danlos syndromes/hypermobility spectrum disorders. *Journal of Personalized Medicine 10*(4), 260. doi:10.3390%2Fjpm10040260.

Casanova, E.L., Sharp, J.L., Edeslon, S.M., Kelly, D.P. & Casanova, M.F. (2018). A cohort study comparing women with autism spectrum disorder with and without generalized joint hypermobility. *Behaviorial Sciences 8*(3), 35. doi:10.3390/bs8030035.

Cascio, C.J., Woynaroski, T., Baranek, G.T. & Wallace, M.T. (2016). Toward an interdisciplinary approach to understanding sensory function in autism spectrum disorder. *Autism Research 9*(9), 920–925. doi:10.1002/aur.1612.

Cassidy, E. (2019). Publisher defends memoir autistic people say depicts abuse of woman's autistic son. The Mighty, 29 September. https://themighty.com/2018/03/autism-uncensored-whitney-ellenby-koehler-books.

Centers for Disease Control and Prevention (2018). Myalgic Encephalomyelitis/ Chronic Fatigue Syndrome: Possible Causes. www.cdc.gov/me-cfs/about/ possible-causes.html.

Cheak-Zamora, N.C., Teti, M., Maurer-Batjer, A. & Koegler, E. (2017). Exploration and comparison of adolescents with autism spectrum disorder and their caregiver's perspectives on transitioning to adult health care and adulthood. *Journal of Pediatric Psychology 42*(9), 1028–1039. doi:10.1093/jpepsy/jsx075.

Chen, I. (2015). Wide awake: Why children with autism struggle with sleep. *Spectrum News*, 7 October. www.spectrumnews.org/features/deep-dive/ wide-awake-why-children-with-autism-struggle-with-sleep.

Chisholm, K., Lin, A., Abu-Akel, A. & Wood, S.J. (2015). The association between autism and schizophrenia spectrum disorders: A review of eight alternate models of co-occurrence. *Neuroscience and Biobehavioral Reviews 55*, 173–183. doi:10.1016/j.neubiorev.2015.04.012.

Chown, N., Robinson, J., Beardon, L., Downing, J. *et al.* (2017). Improving research about us, with us: A draft framework for inclusive autism research. *Disability & Society 32*(5), 720–734. doi:10.1080/09687599.2017.1320273.

Churchard, A., Ryder, M., Greenhill, A. & Mandy, W. (2018). The prevalence of autistic traits in a homeless population. *Autism 23*(3), 665–676. doi:10.1177/1362361318768484.

Clarke, C. (2015). Autism spectrum disorder and amplified pain. *Case Reports in Psychiatry 2015*, 930874. doi:10.1155/2015/930874.

Clesse, C., Lighezzolo-Alnot, J., De Lavergne, S., Hamlin, S. & Scheffler, M. (2018). The evolution of birth medicalisation – A systematic review. *Midwifery 66*, 161–167.

Coleman, V. (1985). *The Story of Medicine*. London: Robert Hale.

Cooper, K., Smith, L.G.E. & Russell, A.J. (2018). Gender identity in autism: Sex differences in social affiliation with gender groups. *Journal of Autism and Development Disorders 48*, 3995–4006. doi:10.1007/s10803-018-3590-1.

Costa, A.P., Steffgen, G. & Samson, A.C. (2017). Expressive incoherence and alexithymia in autism spectrum disorder. *Journal of Autism and Developmental Disorders 47*(6), 1659–1672. doi:10.1007/s10803-017-3073-9.

Coulter, A., Roberts, S. & Dixon, A. (2013). *Delivering Better Services for People with Long-Term Conditions: Building the House of Care*. The King's Fund. www.kingsfund.org.uk/sites/default/files/field/field_publication_file/delivering-better-services-for-people-with-long-term-conditions.pdf.

Cox, D. (2014). Are we ready for a prenatal screening test for autism? *The Guardian*, 14 February. www.theguardian.com/science/blog/2014/may/01/ prenatal-scrrening-test-autism-ethical-implications.

Craig, K.D. (2015). Social communication model of pain. *Pain 156*(7), 1198–1199. doi:10.1097/j.pain.0000000000000185.

Crane, J. (2018). 'Save our NHS': Activism, information-based expertise and the 'new times' of the 1980s. *Contemporary British History 33*(1), 52–74.

Crane, L., Adams, F., Harper, G., Welch, J. & Pellicano, E. (2018). 'Something needs to change': Mental health experiences of young autistic adults in England. *Autism 23*(2), 477–493. doi:10.1177/1362361318757048.

Criado-Perez, C. (2019). *Invisible Women.* London: Chatto & Windus.

Croen, L.A., Zerbo, O., Qian, Y., Massolo, M.L. *et al.* (2015). The health status of adults on the autism spectrum. *Autism 19*(7), 814–823. doi:10.1177/1362361315577517.

Crompton, C.J., Ropar, D., Evans-Williams, C.V.M., Flynn, E.G. & Fletcher-Watson, S. (2020). Autistic peer-to-peer information transfer is highly effective. *Autism 24*(7). doi:10.1177/1362361320919286.

Cummins, C., Pellicano, E. & Crane, L. (2020). Supporting minimally verbal autistic girls with intellectual disabilities through puberty: Perspectives of parents and educators. *Journal of Autism and Developmental Disorders 50*(7), 2439–2448. doi:10.1007/s10803-018-3782-8.

Curcio, F. (1978). Sensorimotor functioning and communication in mute autistic children. *Journal of Autism and Child Schizophrenia 8*(3), 281–292.

Davignon, M.N., Qian, Y., Massolo, M. & Croen, L.A. (2018). Psychiatric and medical conditions in transition-aged individuals with ASD. *Pediatrics 141*(Suppl. 4), S335–345. https://doi.org/10.1542/peds.2016-4300k.

Davis, P., Murtagh, U. & Glaser, D. (2019). 40 years of fabricated or induced illness (FII): Where next for paediatricians? Paper 1: Epidemiology and definition of FII. *Archives of Disease in Childhood 104*, 110–114. https://adc.bmj.com/content/104/2/110.info.

Dear, A. (2019). Meghan Markle: Expert issues high heel warning to Duchess of Sussex as she wears high heels at six months pregnant. Heart, 18 January. www.heart.co.uk/news/royals/meghan-markle/pregnant-high-heels-dangers-duchess-of-sussex.

De Benedictis, S. & Gill, R. (2016). Austerity neoliberalism: A new discursive formation. Open Democracy UK. https://bura.brunel.ac.uk/bitstream/2438/16499/1/Fulltext.pdf.

Delfos, D.M. (2017). *Unravelling Autism: Introduction to Autism with the Socioscheme.* Amsterdam: SWP Publishing.

Delfos, M. (2004). *Children and Behavioural Problems: Anxiety, Aggression, Depression and ADHD – A Biopsychological Model with Guidelines for Diagnostics and Treatment.* London: Jessica Kingsley Publishers.

Delfos, M. (2016). *Wondering about the World: About Autism Spectrum Conditions.* Amsterdam: SWP Publshers.

Department of Health and Social Care (2012). *Long Term Conditions Compendium of Information: Third Edition.* www.gov.uk/government/publications/long-term-conditions-compendium-of-information-third-edition.

Devnani, P.A. & Hegde, A.U. (2015). Autism and sleep disorders. *Journal of Pediatric Neurosciences 10*(4), 304–307. doi:10.4103%2F1817-1745.174438.

Doherty, M. (2023). Weaponized heterogeneity only harms the most vulnerable autistic people. *Spectrum News*, 17 April. www.spectrumnews.org/opinion/viewpoint/weaponized-heterogeneity-only-harms-the-most-vulnerable-autistic-people.

Donohue, M.R., Childs, A.W., Richards, M. & Robins, D.L. (2017). Race influences parent report of concerns about symptoms of autism spectrum disorder. *Autism 23*(1), 100–111. doi:10.1177/1362361317722030.

Donovan, J. (2017). *The Experiences of Autistic Women During Childbirth in an Acute Care Setting.* Doctoral dissertation, Widener University. www.proquest.com/openview/31d16df9cd1317433beb4abb828549b3/1?pq-origsite=gscholar&cbl=18750.

Dooris, M. & Rocca-Ihenacho, L. (2019). Healthy Settings and Birth. In S. Downe & S. Byrom (eds) *Squaring the Circle: Normal Birth Research, Theory and Practice in a Technological Age* (pp.241–250). London: Pinter & Martin.

Doran, G. (1981). There's a S.M.A.R.T. way to write management's goals and objectives. *Management Review 70*(11), 35–36.

Downe, S. & Byrom, S. (2019). *Squaring the Circle: Normal Birth Research, Theory and Practice in a Technological Age.* London: Pinter & Martin.

DuBois, D., Ameis, S.H., Lai, M.-C., Casanova, M.F. & Desarkar, P. (2016). Interoception in autism spectrum disorder: A review. *International Journal of Developmental Neuroscience 52*(1), 104–111. doi:10.1016/j.ijdevneu.2016.05.001.

Dudas, R.B., Lovejoy, C., Cassidy, S., Allison, C., Smith, P. & Baron-Cohen, S. (2017). The overlap between autistic spectrum conditions and borderline personality disorder. *PLoS One 12*(9): e0184447.

Duerden, E.G., Card, D., Roberts, S.W., Mak-Fan, K.M. *et al.* (2013). Self-injurious behaviours are associated with alterations in the somatosensory system in children with autism spectrum disorder. *Brain Structure and Function 219*(4), 1251–1261. doi:10.1007/s00429-013-0562-2.

Durkin, M.S., Maenner, M.J., Baio, J., Christensen, D. *et al.* (2017). Autism spectrum disorder among US children (2002–2010): Socioeconomic, racial, and ethnic disparities. *American Journal of Public Health 107*(11), 1818–1826. doi:10.2105/ajph.2017.304032.

Durman, E. (2023) The metaphor I use to explain autistic shutdown and burnout. The Mighty. Blog post, 21 July. https://themighty.com/topic/autism-spectrum-disorder/autistic-shutdown-disk-defragmentation.

Du Toit, E., Thomas, E., Koen, L., Vythilingum, B. *et al.* (2015). SSRI use in pregnancy: Evaluating the risks and benefits. *South African Journal of Psychiatry 21*(2), a587. https://doi.org/10.4102/sajpsychiatry.v21i2.587.

Dyer, O. (2016). UK junior doctors set for five-day strike action. *Canadian Medical Association Journal 188*(15), E372.

Eaton, J. & Banting, R. (2012). Adult diagnosis of pathological demand avoidance – subsequent care planning. *Journal of Learning Disabilities and Offending Behaviour 3*(3). doi:10.1108/20420921211305891.

Eberjer, J.L, Medland, S.E., van der Werf, J., Gondro, C. *et al.* (2012). Attention deficit hyperactivity disorder in Australian adults: Prevalence, persistence, conduct problems and disadvantage. *PLoS ONE 7*(10), e47404. doi:10.1371/journal.pone.0047404.

ECHR (1953). *European Convention on Human Rights.* www.echr.coe.int/documents/convention_eng.pdf.

Egan, V., Linenberg, O. & O'Nions, E. (2019). The measurement of pathological demand avoidance traits. *Journal of Autism and Developmental Disorders 49*, 481–494. doi:10.1007/s10803-018-3722-7.

Eigsti, I.M. & de Marchena, A. (2017). Perspectives on gesture from autism spectrum disorder: Alterations in timing and function. *Behavioral and Brain Sciences 40*, e53.

Elverdam, B. & Wielandt, H. (1994). The duration of human pregnancy – medical fact or cultural tradition? *International Journal of Prenatal and Perinatal Psychology and Medicine 6*(2), 239–246.

Equality Act (2010). www.legislation.gov.uk/ukpga/2010/15/contents/enacted.

ESNEFT (East Suffolk and North Essex Foundation Trust) (2021). Maternity support plans developed to support women with autism. Press release, 25 January. www.esneft.nhs.uk/maternity-support-plans-developed-to-support-women-with-autism.

Evening Standard (2013). Report to reveal 'shocking' care at Stafford Hospital, 6 February. www.standard.co.uk/news/health/report-to-reveal-shocking-care-at-stafford-hospital-8482627.html.

Failla, M.D., Moana-Filho, E.J., Essick, G.K., Baranek, G.T., Rogers, B.P. & Cascio, C.J. (2017). Initially intact neural responses to pain in autism are diminished during sustained pain. *Autism 22*(6), 669–683. doi:10.1177/1362361317696043.

Faso, D.J., Sasson, N.J. & Pinkham, A.E. (2015). Evaluating posed and evoked facial expressions of emotion from adults with autism spectrum disorder. *Journal of Autism and Developmental Disorders 45*(1), 75–89.

Fidler, R. & Christie, P. (2017). Educational provision and teaching approaches for children with PDA. https://notesonpda.wordpress.com/educational-provision-and-teaching-approaches-for-children-with-pda.

Findon, J., Cadman, T., Stewart, C.S., Woodhouse, E. *et al.* (2016). Screening for co-occurring conditions in adults with autism spectrum disorder using the strengths and difficulties questionnaire: A pilot study. *Autism Research 9*(12), 1353–1363. doi:10.1002/aur.1625.

Flannery, K.A. & Wisner-Carlson, R. (2020). Autism and education. *Child and Adolescent Psychiatry Clinics of North America 29*(2), 319–343. doi:10.1016/j.chc.2019.12.005.

Fletcher-Watson, S., McConnell, F., Manola, E. & McConachie, H. (2014). Interventions based on the Theory of Mind cognitive model for autism spectrum disorder (ASD). *Cochrane Database of Systematic Reviews*, Issue 3. Art. No.: CD008785.

Fletcher-Watson, S. & Happé, F. (2019). *Autism: A New Introduction to Psychological Theory and Current Debate*. London: Routledge/Taylor & Francis Group. doi:10.4324/9781315101699.

Flynn, T.W., Smith, B. & Chou, R. (2011). A reminder that unnecessary imaging may do as much harm as good. *Journal of Orthopaedic and Sports Physical Therapy 41*(11), 838–846. doi:10.2519/jospt.2011.3618.

Fombonne, E. (2009). Epidemiology of pervasive development disorders. *Pediatric Research 65*, 591–598. https://doi.org/10.1203/PDR.0b013e31819e7203.

Fox, D. (2022). Supporting pregnant autistic people. National Autistic Society, 6 October. www.autism.org.uk/advice-and-guidance/professional-practice/pregnant-autistic.

Friedman, E.A. (1954). The graphic analysis of labour. *American Journal of Obstetrics and Gynecology 68*, 1568–1575.

Friedman, E.A. (1955). Primigravid labour: A graphicostatistical analysis. *American Journal of Obstetrics and Gynecology 6*, 567–589.

Frith, U. (1989). Autism and 'Theory of Mind'. In C. Gillberg (ed.) *Diagnosis and Treatment of Autism* (pp.33–52). Boston, MA: Springer.

Frohmader, C. & Ortoleva, S. (2012). The sexual and reproductive rights of women and girls with disabilities. ICPD International Conference on Population and Development Beyond 2014, July 2012. https://ssrn.com/abstract=2444170.

Ganapathy, T. (2015). Tokophobia among first time expectant fathers. *Journal of Depression and Anxiety 3*. doi:10.4172/2167-1044.s3-002.

Garcia, R., Ali, N., Papadopoulos, C. & Randhawa, G. (2015). Specific antenatal interventions for Black, Asian and Minority Ethnic (BAME) pregnant women at high risk of poor birth outcomes in the United Kingdom: A scoping review. *BMC Pregnancy and Childbirth 15*(1). doi:10.1186/s12884-015-0657-2.

Garisto Pfaff, L. (2018). How adults with autism navigate sex on the spectrum. *New Jersey Monthly*, 9 May. https://njmonthly.com/articles/jersey-living/sex-on-the-spectrum.

George, R. & Stokes, M.A. (2017). Gender identity and sexual orientation in autism spectrum disorder. *Autism 22*(8), 970–982. doi:10.1177/1362361317714587.

Gholipour, D. (2018). Schizophrenia prevalence may be threefold higher in people with autism. Spectrum, 21 November. www.spectrumnews.org/news/schizophrenia-prevalence-may-threefold-higher-people-autism.

Gibbs, G. (1988). *Learning by Doing: A Guide to Teaching and Learning Methods.* Oxford: Oxford Polytechnic, Further Education Unit.

Gibert, S.H., DeGrazia, D. & Danis, M. (2017). Ethics of patient activation: Exploring its relation to personal responsibility, autonomy and health disparities. *Journal of Medical Ethics 43*(10), 670–675. doi:10.1136/medethics-2017-104260.

Glasby, J. (2018). Health and social care: What's in a name? *British Medical Journal 360*, k201.

Glidden, D., Bouman, W.P., Jones, B.A. & Arcelus, J. (2016). Gender dysphoria and autism spectrum disorder: A systematic review of the literature. *Sexual Medicine Reviews 4*(1), 3–14. doi:10.1016/j.sxmr.2015.10.003.

Goldacre, A.D., Gray, R. & Goldacre, M.J. (2015). Childbirth in women with intellectual disability: Characteristics of their pregnancies and outcomes in an archived epidemiological dataset. *Journal of Intellectual Disability Research 59*(7), 653–663. doi:10.1111/jir.12169.

Gomer Blog (2014). Study: Length of birth plan correlates to length of C-section scar. GomerBlog, 17 May. https://gomerblog.com/2014/05/birth-plan.

Gore-Langton, E. & Frederickson, N. (2015). Mapping the educational experiences of children with pathological demand avoidance. *JORSEN: Journal of Research in Special Educational Needs 16*(5), 215–298. doi:10.1111/1471-3802.12081.

Gore-Langton, E. & Frederickson, N. (2016). Parents' experiences of professionals' involvement for children with extreme demand avoidance. *International Journal of Developmental Disabilities 64*(1), 16–24. doi:10.1080/20473869.2016.1204743.

Gottfried, R., Lev-Wiesel, R., Hallak, M. & Lang-Franco, N. (2015). Interrelationships between sexual abuse, female sexual function and childbirth. *Midwifery 31*(11), 1087–1095. doi:10.1016/j.midw.2015.07.011.

Grant, A. (2022). CRAE Webinar Series 2022–2023 – Aimee Grant 3/11/2022. YouTube. https://www.youtube.com/watch?v=SilegsmFo6U&t=2s.

Grant, A., Jones, S., Williams, K., Leigh, J. & Brown, A. (2022). Autistic women's views and experiences of infant feeding: A systematic review of qualitative evidence. *Autism 26*(6), 1341-1352.

Grant, L. (2017). Autistic women, pregnancy and motherhood. National Autistic Society, 25 January. https://network.autism.org.uk/knowledge/insight-opinion/autistic-women-pregnancy-and-motherhood.

Grant, S., Norton, S., Weiland, R.F. et al. (2022). Autism and chronic ill health: An observational study of symptoms and diagnoses of central sensitivity syndromes in autistic adults. *Molecular Autism 13*(7).

Gray, C. (2000). *The New Social Stories Book*. Arlington, TX: Future Horizon.

Grice, P. (1991) *Studies in the Way of Words*. Cambridge, MA: Harvard University Press.

Griffin OT (2018). What is tactile defensiveness, or touch sensitivity? www.griffinot.com/what-is-tactile-defensiveness.

Güneş, G. & Karaçam, Z. (2017). The feeling of discomfort during vaginal examination, history of abuse and sexual abuse and post-traumatic stress disorder in women. *Journal of Clinical Nursing 26*(15–16), 2362–2371. doi:10.1111/jocn.13574.

Haddon, M. (2003). *The Curious Incident of the Dog in the Night-Time*. London: Jonathan Cape.

Hadjikhani, N., Zürcher, N.R., Rogier, O., Hippolyte, L. *et al.* (2014). Emotional contagion for pain is intact in autism spectrum disorders. *Translational Psychiatry 4*(1), e343–e343. doi:10.1038/tp.2013.113.

Hahn, S. (2012). Environments and autistic spectrum conditions. *Nursing Times 108*(49), 23–25.

Hakim, A. & Grahame, R. (2003). Joint hypermobility. *Best Practice and Reasearch. Clinical Rheumatology 17*(6), 989–1004.

Hall, J. (2021). Capturing the correct data for births at home. Maternity and Midwifery Forum, June. www.maternityandmidwifery.co.uk/homebirth.

Halliday, J. (2018). NHS trust fined £2m for Connor Sparrowhawk and Teresa Colvin deaths. *The Guardian*, 26 March. www.theguardian.com/society/2018/mar/26/nhs-trust-fined-2m-over-death-of-teenager-connor-sparrowhawk.

Ham, C. (2017). Political crisis in the NHS. The King's Fund, 17 January. www.kingsfund.org.uk/publications/articles/political-crisis-nhs.

Hambrook, D., Tchanturia, K., Schmidt, U., Russell, T. & Treasure, J. (2008). Empathy, systemizing, and autistic traits in anorexia nervosa: A pilot study. *British Journal of Clinical Psychology 47*(3), 335–339. doi:10.1348/014466507x272475.

Hampton, S., Allison, C., Baron-Cohen, S. & Holt, R. (2022). Autistic people's perinatal experiences I: A survey of pregnancy experiences. *Journal of Autism and Developmental Disorders*. doi:10.1007/s10803-022-05754-1.

Handley, E. (2016). Richard's story: Unmanaged constipation in people with learning disabilities. King's Health Partners, 10 October. www.kingshealthpartners.org/latest/739-richards-story-unmanaged-constipation-in-people-with-learning-disabilities.

Hanley, M., Riby, D.M., Carty, C., Melaugh McAteer, A., Kennedy, A. & McPhillips, M. (2015). The use of eye-tracking to explore social difficulties in cognitively able students with autism spectrum disorder: A pilot investigation. *Autism 19*(7), 868–873. doi:10.1177/1362361315580767.

Haque, M. (2019). Importance of empathy among medical doctors to ensure high-quality healthcare level. *Advances in Human Biology 9*(2), 104–107. doi:10.4103/AIHB.AIHB_44_18.

Harmens, M., Sedgewick, F. & Hobson, H. (2022). Autistic women's diagnostic experiences: Interactions with identity and impacts on well-being. *Women's Health*. doi:10.1177/17455057221137477.

Harrison, A.J., Long, K.A., Tommet, D.C. & Jones, R.N. (2017). Examining the role of race, ethnicity, and gender on social and behavioral ratings within the Autism Diagnostic Observation Schedule. *Journal of Autism and Developmental Disorders 47*(9), 2770–2782. doi:10.1007/s10803-017-3176-3.

Hatfield, T.R., Brown, R.F., Giummarra, M.J. & Lenggenhager, B. (2019). Autism spectrum disorder and interoception: Abnormalities in global integration? *Autism 23*(1), 212–222. doi:10.1177/1362361317738392.

Havercamp, S.M., Ratliff-Schaub, K., Macho, P.N., Johnson, C.N. Bush, K.L. & Souders, H.T. (2016). Preparing tomorrow's doctors to care for patients with autism spectrum disorder. *Intellectual and Developmental Disabilities 54*(3), 202–216. doi:10.1352/1934-9556-54.3.202.

Hayward, S.M., McVilly, K.R. & Stokes, M.A. (2018). Challenges for females with high functioning autism in the workplace: A systematic review. *Disability and Rehabilitation 40*(3), 249–258. doi:10.1080/09638288.2016.1254284.

Hazard, L. (2019). *Hard Pushed: A Midwife's Story*. New York, NY: Random House.

He, Y. & Kim, P.Y. (2022). Allodynia. StatPearls. Treasure Island, FL: StatPearls Publishing.

Healthcare Quality Improvement Partnership (2019). *The Learning Disability Mortality Review (LeDeR) Programme: Annual Report 2018*. www.hqip.org.uk/wp-content/uploads/2019/05/LeDeR-Annual-Report-Final-21-May-2019.pdf.

Healthcare Quality Improvement Partnership (2020). *The Learning Disability Mortality Review (LeDeR) Programme: Annual Report 2019*. www.bristol.ac.uk/media-library/sites/sps/leder/LeDeR_2019_annual_report_FINAL2.pdf.

Henry, K. (2017). Empowering women with autism. *Midwifery Matters* 155, 10–11. Northumberland: Association of Radical Midwives.

Henry, K. (2022). Addressing inequity and inequality within maternity services for autistic women. Maternity & Midwife Forum. www.maternityandmidwifery.co.uk/addressing-inequity-and-inequality-within-maternity-services-for-autistic-women.

Henry, K. (2023). Providing accessible healthcare for autistic women. *The Practising Midwife 26*(2), 37–41. doi:10.55975/VGTY3495.

Heyworth, M., Brett, S., den Houting, J., Magiati, I. *et al.* (2023). 'I'm the family ringmaster and juggler': Autistic parents' experiences of parenting during the COVID-19 pandemic. *Autism in Adulthood 5*(1), 24–36. doi:10.1089/aut.2021.0097.

Hildingsson, I., Rubertsson, C., Karlström, A. & Haines, H. (2018). Caseload midwifery for women with fear of birth is a feasible option. *Sexual & Reproductive Healthcare 16*, 50–55. doi:10.1016/j.srhc.2018.02.006.

Hill, A. (2017). Mothers with autism: 'I mothered my children in a very different way'. *The Guardian*, 20 September. www.theguardian.com/lifeandstyle/2017/apr/15/women-autistic-mothers-undiagnosed-children.

Hill, M. (2019a). *Give Birth Like a Feminist*. London: HarperCollins.

Hill, M. (2019b). 'Shut up, close your mouth and push.' We need to talk about women's experiences of obstetric violence. MamaMia, 28 September. www.mamamia.com.au/violence-and-childbirth.

Hillary, A. (2013). Autistic and pregnant. Yes, That Too. Blog post, 5 February. https://yesthattoo.blogspot.com/2013/02/autistic-and-pregnant.html.

Hirvikoski, T., Mittendorf-Rutz, E., Boman, M., Larsson, H., Lichtenstein, P. & Bölte, S. (2016). Premature mortality in autism spectrum disorder. *British Journal of Psychiatry 208*(3), 232–238. doi:10.1192/bjp.bp.114.160192.

Historic England (2022). The age of the madhouse – Home of the well-attired ploughman. https://historicengland.org.uk/research/inclusive-heritage/disability-history/1660-1832/the-age-of-the-madhouse.

Hoang, S. (2014). Pregnancy and anxiety. *International Journal of Childbirth Education 29*(1), 67–70.

Hodgetts, S., Richards, K. & Park, E. (2017). Preparing for the future: Multistakeholder perspectives on autonomous goal setting for adolescents with autism spectrum disorders. *Disability and Rehabilitation 40*(20), 2372–2379. doi:10.1080/09638288.2017.1334836.

Hoekstra, R.A., Girma, F., Tekola, B. & Yenus, Z. (2018). Nothing about us without us: The importance of local collaboration and engagement in the global study of autism. *BJPsych International 15*(2), 40–43. doi:10.1192/bji.2017.26.

Hollander, M.H., van Hastenburg, E., van Dillen, J., van Pampus, M.G., de Miranda, E. & Stamrood, C.A.I. (2017). Preventing traumatic childbirth experiences: 2192 women's perceptions and views. *Archives of Women's Mental Health 20*(4), 515–523. doi:10.1007/s00737-017-0729-6.

Home Office (2023). Domestic abuse: Draft statutory guidance framework. www.gov.uk/government/consultations/domestic-abuse-act-statutory-guidance/domestic-abuse-draft-statutory-guidance-framework.

Howick, J. & Rees, S. (2017). Overthrowing barriers to empathy in healthcare: Empathy in the age of the Internet. *Journal of the Royal Society of Medicine 110*(9), 352–357. doi:10.1177/0141076817714443.

HSIB (Healthcare Safety Investigation Branch) (2022). What we investigate. www.hsib.org.uk/what-we-do/maternity-investigations/what-we-investigate.

Hull, L., Petrides, K.V., Allison, C.A., Smith, P. *et al.* (2017). 'Putting on my best normal': Social camouflaging in adults with autism spectrum condition. *Journal of Autism and Developmental Disorders 47*, 2519–2534. doi:10.1007/s10803-017-3166-5.

Human Rights Act 1998 (1998). www.legislation.gov.uk/ukpga/1998/42/contents.

Hwang, S.K. & Heslop, P. (2023). Autistic parents' personal experiences of parenting and support: Messages from an online focus group. *British Journal of Social Work 53*(1), 276–295. doi:10.1093/bjsw/bcac133.

Iacobucci, G. (2017a). NHS in 2017: A service under pressure. *BMJ 356*, i6691. doi:10.1136/bmj.i6691.

Iacobucci, G. (2017b). NHS in 2017: Keeping pace with society. *BMJ 356*, i6738. doi:10.1136/bmj.i6738.

Iacobucci, G. (2017c). NHS in 2017: The long arm of government. *BMJ 356*, j41. doi:10.1136/bmj.j41.

Iacobucci, G. (2017d). NHS in 2017: A medical profession in step with today's NHS? *BMJ 356*, j204. doi:10.1136/bmj.j204.

Iacobucci, G. (2017e). NHS in 2017: Where next? *BMJ 356*, j331. doi:10.1136/bmj.j331.

Iles, J., Slade, P. & Spiby, H. (2011). Posttraumatic stress symptoms and postpartum depression in couples after childbirth: the role of partner support and attachment. *Journal of Anxiety Disorders 25*(4), 520–530. doi:10.1016/j.janxdis.2010.12.006.

Inglis, C., Sharman, R. & Reed, R. (2016). Paternal mental health following perceived traumatic childbirth. *Midwifery 41*, 125–131. doi:10.1016/j.midw.2016.08.008.

International Baby Foods Action Network (IBFAN) (2020). IBFAN Network in action. www.IBFAN.org/all-about-IBFAN.

International Society for Autism Research (2019). *Annual Meeting: Program Book: May 1–4 Montreal, Canada.* https://cdn.ymaws.com/www.autism-insar.org/resource/resmgr/files/2019_annual_meeting/2019insar_program_bk.pdf.

Isaksen, J., Bryn, V., Diseth, T.H., Heiberg, A., Schjølberg, S. & Skjedal, O.H. (2012). Children with autism spectrum disorders – the importance of medical investigations. *European Journal of Paediatric Neurology 17*(1), P68–76. doi:10.1016/j.ejpn.2012.08.004.

Jacobs, L.A., Rachlin, K., Erickson-Schroth, L. & Janssen, A. (2014). Gender dysphoria and co-occurring autism spectrum disorders: Review, case examples, and treatment considerations. *LGBT Health 1*(4), 277–282. doi:10.1089/lgbt.2013.0045.

Janssen, A., Huang, H. & Duncan, C. (2016). Gender variance among youth with autism spectrum disorders: A retrospective chart review. *Transgender Health 1*(1), 63–68. doi:10.1089/trgh.2015.0007.

Jarrett, S. (2012). A history of disability: From 1050 to the present day. Historic England. https://historicengland.org.uk/research/inclusive-heritage/disability-history.

Jennings, L., Goût, B. and Whittaker, P.J. (2022). Gender inclusive language on public-facing maternity services websites in England. *British Journal of Midwifery 30*(4).

Jones, B., Horton, T. & Home, J. (2022). Strengthening NHS management and leadership. The Health Foundation, 26 February. www.health.org.uk/publications/long-reads/strengthening-nhs-management-and-leadership.

Jones, E. (2019). Given Greta Thunberg's bullying, is it any wonder so few women share that they're autistic? *HuffPost*, 2 September. www.huffingtonpost.co.uk/entry/greta-thunberg-autism_uk_5d6d1930e4b0cdfe0573695a.

Jones-Berry, S. (2017). Student drop-out rates put profession at further risk. *Nursing Standard 32*(2), 12–13. doi:10.7748/ns.32.2.12.s13.

Jo's Cervical Cancer Trust (2019). Let's talk about…accessing smear tests when you have a physical disability. Blog post, 23 January. www.jostrust.org.uk/about-us/news-and-blog/blog/lets-talk-about-it/smear-tests-physical-disability.

Källén, B., Finnstrom, O., Nygren, K.G. & Olausson, P.O. (2013). Maternal and fetal factors which affect fetometry: Use of vitro fertilization and birth register data. *European Journal of Obstetrics, Gynaecology and Reproductive Biology 170*(2), 372–376.

Kanakaris, N.K., Roberts, C.S. & Giannoudis, P.V. (2011). Pregnancy-related pelvic girdle pain: An update. *BMC Medicine 9*, 15. doi:10.1186/1741-7015-9-15.

Kargas, N., Harley, K.M., Roberts, A. & Sharman, S. (2019). Prevalence of clinical autistic traits within a homeless population: Barriers to accessing homeless services. *Journal of Social Distress and the Homeless 28*(2), 90–95. doi:10.1080/10530789.2019.1607139.

Karthikeyan, A. & Venkat-Raman, N. (2018). Hypermobile Ehlers–Danlos syndrome and pregnancy. *Obstetric Medicine 11*(3), 104–109. doi:10.1177/1753495x18754577.

Kaufman, S.B. (2020). Autistic people make great social partners if you actually give them a chance. *Scientific American*, 9 March. https://blogs.scientificamerican.com/beautiful-minds/autistic-people-make-great-social-partners-if-you-actually-give-them-a-chance.

Kay, A. (2018). *This Is Going to Hurt: Secret Diaries of a Junior Doctor.* London: Pan Macmillan.

Kay, L. (2019). Respectful maternity care: Mapping current global initiatives designed to achieve a positive experience of childbirth, reduce interventions without clinical benefit or increase access to high quality maternity care. 14th International Normal Labour and Birth Conference, 17–19 June, Grange-over Sands, Cumbria.

Kennedy, R., Binns, F., Brammer, A., Grant, J., Bowen, J. & Morgan, R. (2016). Continuous service quality improvement and change management for children and young people with autism and their families: A model for change. *Comprehensive Child and Adolescent Nursing 39*(3), 192–214. doi:10.1080/2469 4193.2016.1178357.

Kiep, M. & Spek, A.A. (2017). Executive functioning in men and women with an autism spectrum disorder. *Autism Research 10*(5), 940–948. doi:10.1002/ aur.1721.

Kilbaugh, T.J., Friess, S.H., Raghupathi, R. & Huh, J.W. (2010). Sedation and analgesia in children with developmental disabilities and neuroligic disorders. *International Journal of Pediatrics 2010*, 189142. doi:10.1155/2010/189142.

Kim, C. (2014a). Honoring our choices. Musings of an Aspie. Blog post, 17 April. https://musingsofanaspie.com/2014/04/17/honoring-our-choices/#more-2121kim.

Kim, C. (2014b). Autistic motherhood: Honoring our personal choices. Autism Women's Network AWN. Blog post, 17 April. https://awnnetwork.org/ autistic-motherhood-honoring-our-personal-choices.

Kimmel, M., Ferguson, E., Zerwas, S., Bulik, C. & Meltzer-Brody, S. (2015). Obstetric and gynecologic problems associated with eating disorders. *International Journal of Eating Disorders 49*(3), 260–275. doi:10.1002/eat.22483.

King, S. (2019). Personal stories: Sara King. Autistica. https://www.autistica.org. uk/get-involved/my-autism-story/sara-king.

King's Fund (2012). Long-term conditions and multi-morbidity. www.kingsfund. org.uk/projects/time-think-differently/trends-disease-and-disability-long-term-conditions-multi-morbidity.

King's Fund (2018). The NHS at 70. www.kingsfund.org.uk/projects/NHS70/ research-group.

Kinsey Institute (2023). The Kinsey Scale. https://kinseyinstitute.org/research/ publications/kinsey-scale.php.

Kirkovski, M., Enticott, P.G. & Fitzgerald, P.B. (2013). A review of the role of female gender in autism spectrum disorders. *Journal of Autism and Developmental Disorders 43*(11), 2584–2603.

Kitzinger, S. (1991). *The Midwife Challenge*, 2nd edn. London: Pandora Press.

Knight, M., Bunch, K., Patel, R., Shakespere, J. *et al.* (eds) (2022). *Saving Lives: Improving Mothers' Care: Lessons Learned to Inform Maternity Care from the UK and Ireland Confidential Enquiries into Maternal Deaths and Morbidity 2018–20.* Oxford: MBRRACE-UK.

Koblinsky, M., Moyer, C.A., Calvert, C., Campbell, J. *et al.* (2016). Quality of maternity care for every woman, everywhere: A call to action. *Lancet 388*(10057), 2307–2320. doi:10.1016/s0140-6736(16)31333-2.

Kong, X., Liu, J., Chien, T., Batalden, M. & Hirsh, D.A. (2019). A systematic network of autism primary care services (SYNAPSE): A model of coproduction for the management of autism spectrum disorder. *Journal of Autism and Developmental Disorders.* doi:10.1007/s10803-019-03922-4.

Koo, S., Gaul, K., Rivera, S., Pan, T. & Fong, D. (2018). Wearable technology design for autism spectrum disorders. *Archives of Design Research*. doi:10.15187/adr.2018.02.31.1.37.

Krahn, T.M. & Fenton, A. (2012). The extreme male brain theory of autism and the potential adverse effects for boys and girls with autism. *Journal of Bioethical Inquiry 9*(1), 93–103. doi:10.1007/s11673-011-9350-y.

Labor, S. & Maguire, S. (2008). The pain of labour. *Reviews in Pain 2*(2), 15–19. doi:10.3389/fpsyt.2018.00656.

Lahiri, D.K., Sokol, D.K., Erickson, C., Ray, B., Ho, C.Y. & Maloney, B. (2013). Autism as early neurodevelopmental disorder: Evidence for an sAPPα-mediated anabolic pathway. *Frontiers in Cellular Neuroscience 7*. doi:10.3389/fncel.2013.00094.

Lai, M., Baron-Cohen, S. & Buxbaum, J.D. (2015). Understanding autism in the light of sex/gender. *Molecular Autism 6*(1). doi:10.1186/s13229-015-0021-4.

Lambert, M. (2017). Austerity has trampled over disabled people's rights. But the UK won't admit it. *The Guardian*, 4 September. www.theguardian.com/commentisfree/2017/sep/04/austerity-disabled-people-rights-uk-un-government.

Landa, R.J. (2008). Diagnosis of autism spectrum disorders in the first 3 years of life. *Nature Clinical Practice Neurology 4*, 138–147.

Lavender, T., Cuthbert, A. & Smyth, R.M. (2018). Effect of partograph use on outcomes for women in spontaneous labour at term and their babies. *Cochrane Database of Systematic Reviews 8*(8), CD005461. doi: 10.1002/14651858.

Lavender, T., Hart, A. & Smyth, R.M.D. (2008). Effect of partogram use on outcomes for women in spontaneous labour at term. *Cochrane Database of Systematic Reviews 7*, CD005461. doi:10.1002/14651858.CD005461.pub4.

Leap. N. & Hunter, B (2013). *The Midwife's Tale*. Barnsley: Pen and Sword History.

Lee, P. (2007). The Social Construction of Disability and Motherhood. In S. McKay-Moffat (ed.) *Disability in Pregnancy and Childbirth* (pp.1–18). London: Churchill Livingstone Elsevier.

Leeds and York Partnership NHS Foundation Trust (2023). Easy on the i. www.learningdisabilityservice-leeds.nhs.uk/easy-on-the-i.

Lemon, J.M., Gargaro, B., Enticott, P.G. & Rinehart, N.J. (2011). Executive functioning in autism spectrum disorders: A gender comparison of response inhibition. *Journal of Autism and Developmental Disorders 41*(3), 352–356. doi:10.1007/s10803-010-1039-2.

Li, C., Schaefer, M., Gray, C., Yang, Y. *et al.* (2017). Sensitivity to isoflurane anesthesia increases in autism spectrum disorder *Shank3+/Δc* mutant mouse model. *Neurotoxicology and Teratology 60*, 69–74. doi:10.1016/j.ntt.2016.11.002.

Lokugamage, A.U. & Pathberiya, S.D. (2017). Human rights in childbirth, narratives and restorative justice: A review. *Reproductive Health 14*(1). doi:10.1186/s12978-016-0264-3.

Loomes, G. (2018). Researching about us without us: Exploring research participation and the politics of disability rights in the context of the Mental Capacity Act 2005. *Journal of Medical Ethics 44*(6), 424–427. doi:10.1136/medethics-2016-104129.

Loomes, R., Hull, L. & Mandy, W.P. (2017). What is the male-to-female ratio in autism spectrum disorder? A systematic review and meta-analysis. *Journal of the American Academy of Child & Adolescent Psychiatry 56*(6), 466–474. doi:10.1016/j.jaac.2017.03.013.

Lucarelli, L., Ammaniti, M., Porreca, A. & Simonelli, A. (2017). Infantile anorexia and co-parenting: A pilot study on mother–father–child triadic interactions during feeding and play. *Frontiers in Psychology 8*. doi:10.3389/fpsyg.2017.00376.

Lum, M., Garnett, M. & O'Connor, E. (2014). Health communication: A pilot study comparing perceptions of women with and without high functioning autism spectrum disorder. *Research in Autism Spectrum Disorders 8*(12), 1713–1721. doi:10.1016/j.rasd.2014.09.009.

Lyndon, A., Johnson, M.C., Bingham, D., Napolitano, P.G. *et al.* (2015). Transforming communication and safety culture in intrapartum care: A multi-organization blueprint. *Journal of Midwifery & Women's Health 60*(3), 237–243. doi:10.1111/jmwh.12235.

Macdonald, S. & Magill-Cuerden, J. (2012). *Mayes' Midwifery*, 14th edn. London: Bailliere Tindall Elsevier.

MacDonald, T., Noel-Weiss, J., West, D., Walks, M, *et al.* (2016). Transmasculine individuals' experiences with lactation, chestfeeding, and gender identity: A qualitative study. *BMC Pregnancy and Childbirth 16*(1). doi:10.1186/s12884-016-0907-y.

Macias, K. (2018). Black Maternal Health Week addresses deadly disparities in health care for black women and babies. Daily Kos, 13 April. www.dailykos.com/stories/2018/4/13/1756853/-Black-Maternal-Health-Week-addresses-deadly-disparities-in-health-care-for-black-women-and-babies.

Maddox, B.B. & White, S.W. (2015). Comorbid social anxiety disorder in adults with autism spectrum disorder. *Journal of Autism and Developmental Disorders 45*(12). doi:10.1007/s10803-015-2531-5.

Madra, M., Ringel, R. & Margolis, K.G. (2020). Gastrointestinal Issues and Autism Spectrum Disorder. *Child and Adolescent Psychiatric Clinics of North America 29*(3), 501–513.

Mandavilli, A. (2015). The lost girls: Misdiagnosed, misunderstood or missed altogether, many women with autism struggle to get the help they need. *Spectrum News*, 19 October. www.spectrumnews.org/features/deep-dive/the-lost-girls.

Mandell, D. (2018). Dying before their time: Addressing premature mortality among autistic people. *Autism 22*(3), 234–235. doi:10.1177/1362361318764742.

Mandy, W. & Tchanturia, K. (2015). Do women with eating disorders who have social and flexibility difficulties really have autism? A case series. *Molecular Autism 6*(1). doi:10.1186/2040-2392-6-6.

Mankowitz, S.K.W., Gonzalez Fiol, A. & Smiley, R. (2016). Failure to extend epidural labor analgesia for cesarean delivery anesthesia: A focused review. *Anesthesia and Analgesia 123*(5), 1174–1180.

Mannion, A. & Leader, G. (2013). Comorbidity in autism spectrum disorder: A literature review. *Research in Autism Spectrum Disorders 7*(12), 1595–1616. doi:10.1016/j.rasd.2013.09.006.

Marriott, E., Stacey, J., Hewitt, O.M. & Verkuijl, N.E. (2022). Parenting an autistic child: Experiences of parents with significant autistic traits. *Journal of Autism and Developmental Disorders 52*(7), 3182–3193. doi:10.1007/s10803-021-05182-7.

Maslow, A.H. (1943). A theory of human motivation. *Psychological Review 50*(4), 370–396. doi:10.1037/h0054346.

Mason, D., Ingham, B., Urbanowicz, A., Michael, C., *et al.* (2019). A systematic review of what barriers and facilitators prevent and enable physical healthcare services for autistic adults. *Journal of Autism and Developmental Disorders 49*(8), 3387–3400. doi:10.1007/s10803-019-04049-2.

Maternal Mental Health Alliance (2018). *Wales Perinatal Mental Health is Everyone's Business*. London: Maternal Mental Health Alliance. https://maternalmentalhealthalliance.org/wp-content/uploads/Wales-Perinatal-Mental-Health-Briefing.pdf.

Matson, J.L. & Cervantes, P.E. (2014). Commonly studied comorbid psychopathologies among persons with autism spectrum disorder. *Research in Developmental Disabilities 35*(5), 952–962. https://doi.org/10.1016/j.ridd.2014.02.012.

Matthews-King, A. (2017). Landmark study links Tory austerity to 120,000 excess deaths. *The Independent*, 16 November. www.independent.co.uk/news/health/tory-austerity-deaths-study-report-people-die-social-care-government-policy-a8057306.html.

Maxwell, J., Watts Betser, J. & David, D. (2007). *A Health Handbook for Women with Disabilities*. Berkeley, CA: Hesperian.

May, J., Williams, A., Cloke, P. & Cherry, L. (2019). Welfare convergence, bureaucracy, and moral distancing at the food bank. *Antipode 51*(4), 1251–1275. doi:10.1111/anti.12531.

Mazefsky, C.A., Herrington, J., Siegel, M., Scarpa, A. *et al.* (2013). The role of emotion regulation in autism spectrum disorder. *Journal of the American Academy of Child & Adolescent Psychiatry 52*(7), 679–688. https://doi.org/10.1016/j.jaac.2013.05.006.

MBRRACE-UK (Mothers and Babies Reducing Risk through Audits and Confidential Enquiries across the UK) (2018a). Saving lives, improving mothers' care. www.npeu.ox.ac.uk/assets/downloads/mbrrace-uk/reports/MBRRACE-UK%20Maternal%20Report%202018%20-%20Web%20Version.pdf.

MBRRACE-UK (2018b). Perinatal Mortality Surveillance report for births in 2016. www.npeu.ox.ac.uk/mbrrace-uk/reports/perinatal-mortality-surveillance#perinatal-mortality-surveillance-report-for-births-in-2016.

MBRRACE-UK (2021). *Saving Lives: Improving Mothers Care – Lay Summary 2021*. www.npeu.ox.ac.uk/assets/downloads/mbrrace-uk/reports/maternal-report-2021/MBRRACE-UK_Maternal_Report_2021_-_Lay_Summary_v10.pdf.

McCann, L. (2021). Autism and spoon theory. EdPsychEd, 6 April. www.edpsyched.co.uk/blog/autism-spoon-theory.

McCauley, M., Actis Danna, V., Mrema, D. & Van den Broek, N. (2018). 'We know it's labour pain, so we don't do anything': Healthcare provider's knowledge and attitudes regarding the provision of pain relief during labour and after childbirth. *BMC Pregnancy and Childbirth 18*(1). doi:10.1186/s12884-018-2076-7.

McCluskey, L. (2017). McCluskey: Humiliated Hunt should be packing his bags over NHS crisis. LabourList, 9 January. https://labourlist.org/2017/01/mccluskey-humiliated-hunt-should-pack-his-bags-over-nhs-crisis.

McDonnell, C.G. & DeLucia, E.A. (2021). Pregnancy and parenthood among autistic adults: Implications for advancing maternal health and parental well-being. *Autism in Adulthood 3*(1), 100–115. doi:10.1089%2Faut.2020.0046.

McGonigle, J.J., Venkat, A., Beresford, C., Campbell, T.P. & Gabriels, R.L. (2014). Management of agitation in individuals with autism spectrum disorders in the emergency department. *Child and Adolescent Psychiatric Clinics 23*(1), 83–95. doi:10.1016/j.chc.2013.08.003.

McGrath, L., Griffin, V. & Mundy, E. (2016). The psychological impact of austerity: A briefing paper. *Educational Psychology Research and Practice 2*(2), 46–57.

McKay, M. (2020). The energy accounting activity for autism. Medium, 29 January. https://medium.com/age-of-awareness/the-energy-accounting-activity-for-autism-3a245e34bdfb.

Meier, S.M., Petersen, L., Schendel, D.E., Mattheisen, M., Mortensen, P.B. & Mors, O. (2015). Obsessive-compulsive disorder and autism spectrum disorders: Longitudinal and offspring risk. *PLoS ONE 10*(11), e0141703. doi:10.1371/journal.pone.0141703.

Messmer, R.L., Nader, R. & Craig, K.D. (2008). Brief report: Judging pain intensity in children with autism undergoing venepuncture: the influence of facial activity. *Journal of Autism and Developmental Disorders 38*(7), 1391–1394.

Milner, V., McIntosh, H., Colvert, E. & Happé, F. (2019). A qualitative exploration of the female experience of autism spectrum disorder (ASD). *Journal of Autism and Developmental Disorders 49*, 2289–2402. doi:10.1007/s10803-019-03906-4.

Milton, D.E.M. (2012). On the ontological status of autism: The 'double empathy' problem. *Disability & Society 27*(6), 883–887. doi:10.1080/09687599.2012.710008.

Milton, D.E.M. (2017). *A Mismatch of Salience: Explorations of the Nature of Autism from Theory to Practice*. Shoreham-by-Sea: Pavilion.

Milton, D.E.M., Ridout, S., Kourti, M., Loomes, G. & Martin, N. (2019). A critical reflection on the development of the Participatory Autism Research Collective (PARC). *Tizard Learning Disability Review 24*(2), 82–89. doi:10.1108/tldr-09-2018-0029.

Mind (2015). *Supporting People Living with Autism Spectrum Disorder and Mental Health Problems: A Guide for Practitioners and Providers*. London: Mind. www.mind.org.uk/media-a/4400/autism-guide-web-version.pdf

Mind (2023). Dissociation and dissociative disorders. www.mind.org.uk/information-support/types-of-mental-health-problems/dissociation-and-dissociative-disorders/about-dissociation.

Minshawi, N., Hurwitz, S., Fodstad, J., Biebl, S., Morris, D. & McDougle, C. (2014). The association between self-injurious behaviors and autism spectrum disorders. *Psychology Research and Behavior Management 125*. doi:10.2147/prbm.s44635.

Mitchell, G. (2019). NMC suspends three nurses in Whorlton Hall abuse probe. 27 June 2019. www.nursingtimes.net/news/professional-regulation/nmc-suspends-three-nurses-in-whorlton-hall-abuse-probe-27-06-2019.

Mitchell, S. & Schlesinger, M. (2005). Managed care and gender disparities in problematic health care experiences. *Health Services Research 40*(5 pt 1), 1489–1513. doi:10.1111%2Fj.1475-6773.2005.00422.x.

Mitra, M., Manning, S.E. & Lu, E. (2012). Physical abuse around the time of pregnancy among women with disabilities. *Maternal and Child Health Journal 16*(4), 802–806. doi:10.1007/s10995-011-0784-y.

Mitra, M., Parish, S.L., Clements, K.M., Xiaohui, C. and Diop, H. (2015). Pregnancy outcomes among women with intellectual and developmental disabilities. *American Journal of Preventive Medicine 48*(3), 300–308. doi:10.1016/j.jpsychores.2012.07.010.

Mogensen, L. & Mason, J. (2015). The meaning of a label for teenagers negotiating identity: Experiences with autism spectrum disorder. *Sociology of Health and Illness 37*(2), 255–269. doi:10.1111/1467-9566.12208.

Moloney, S. & Gair, S. (2015). Empathy and spiritual care in midwifery practice: Contributing to women's enhanced birth experiences. *Women and Birth 28*(4), 323–328. doi:10.1016/j.wombi.2015.04.009.

Moore, D.J. (2014). Acute pain experience in individuals with autism spectrum disorders: A review. *Autism 19*(4), 387–399. doi:10.1177/1362361314527839.

Morgan, H. (2019). The autistic birth experience – a systematic review and data report. MSc thesis (unpublished), Autism and Related Conditions, Swansea University.

Moseley, R.L., Mohr, B., Lombardo, M.V., Baron-Cohen, S. et al. (2013). Brain and behavioral correlates of action semantic deficits in autism. *Frontiers in Human Neuroscience 7*(725).

Nagle, A. & Samari, G. (2021). State-level structural sexism and caesarean sections in the United States. *Social Science and Medicine 289*, 114406. doi:10.1016/j. socscimed.2021.114406.

NAS (National Autistic Society) (2014). *Diverse Perspectives: The Challenges for Families Affected by Autism from Black, Asian and Minority Ethnic Communities.* London: NAS. https://positiveaboutautism.co.uk/uploads/9/7/4/5/97454370/nas-diverse-perspectives-report-1.pdf.

NAS (2021a). School report 2021. https://s2.chorus-mk.thirdlight.com/file/24/0HTGORW0HHJnx_c0HLZm0HWvpWc/NAS-Education-Report-2021-A4%20%281%29.pdf.

NAS (2021b). Eating disorders. www.autism.org.uk/advice-and-guidance/topics/mental-health/eating-disorders.

NAS (2023). Autism, pregnancy and childbirth. www.autism.org.uk/advice-and-guidance/topics/physical-health/pregnancy-and-childbirth.

Nathenson, R.A. & Zablotsky, B. (2017). The transition to the adult health care system among youths with autism spectrum disorder. *Psychiatric Services 68*(7), 735–738. doi:10.1176/appi.ps.201600239.

National Institute for Health and Care Excellence (NICE) (2009). Depression in adults: recognition and management. Clinical guideline [CG90]. www.nice. org.uk/Guidance/CG90.

National Institute for Health and Care Excellence (NICE) (2011). Generalised anxiety disorder and panic disorder in adults: management. Clinical guideline [CG113]. www.nice.org.uk/Guidance/CG113.

National Institute for Health and Care Excellence (NICE) (2017). *Intrapartum Care for Healthy Women and Babies.* London: NICE.

National Institute for Health and Care Excellence (NICE) (2019). Intrapartum care for women with existing medical conditions or obstetric complications and their babies NICE guideline [NG121]. www.nice.org.uk/guidance/ng121.

National Institute for Health and Care Excellence (NICE) (2021). Antenatal care. Clinical guideline [NG201]. www.nice.org.uk/guidance/ng201.

Newcastle upon Tyne Hospitals NHS Foundation Trust (2023). Drug and alcohol midwives. www.newcastle-hospitals.nhs.uk/services/maternity/during-pregnancy/specialist-midwives/drug-and-alcohol-midwives.

Newry SureStart (2023). Midwifery. https://newrysurestart.org/midwifery-2.

Newschaffer, C.J. (2017). Trends in autism spectrum disorders: The interaction of time, group-level socioeconomic status, and individual-level race/ethnicity. *American Journal of Public Health 107*(11), 1698–1699. doi:10.2105/ajph.2017.304085.

Newson, E., Le Maréchal, K. & David, C. (2003). Pathological demand avoidance syndrome: A necessary distinction within the pervasive developmental disorders. *Archives of Disease in Childhood 88*, 595–600.

NHS (2022). NHS Maternity Statistics, England, 2021–2022. https://digital.nhs.uk/ data-and-information/publications/statistical/nhs-maternity-statistics/2021-22/ deliveries---2022-hes.

NHS England (2016). *National Maternity Review: Better Births: Improving Outcomes of Maternity Services in England*. London: NHS England. www.england.nhs.uk/ wp-content/uploads/2016/02/national-maternity-review-report.pdf.

NHS England (2019a). GP Patient Survey 2019. www.england.nhs.uk/ statistics/2019/07/11/gp-patient-survey-2019.

NHS England (2019b). *Saving Babies' Lives Version Two: A Care Bundle for Reducing Perinatal Mortality*. www.england.nhs.uk/wp-content/uploads/2019/07/ saving-babies-lives-care-bundle-version-two-v5.pdf.

NHS England (2021). *Delivering Continuity of Carer at Full Scale: Guidance on Planning, Implementation and Monitoring 2021/2022*. London: NHS England. www. england.nhs.uk/wp-content/uploads/2021/10/B0961_Delivering-midwifery-continuity-of-carer-at-full-scale.pdf.

NHS Leicestershire Partnership (2023). Autism and mindfulness. www.leicspart. nhs.uk/autism-space/health-and-lifestyle/autism-and-mindfulness.

Nicolaidis, C., Kripke, C.C. & Raymaker, D. (2014). Primary care for adults on the autism spectrum. *Medical Clinics of North America 98*(5), 1169–1191. doi:10.1016/j.mcna.2014.06.011.

Nicolaidis, C. & Raymaker, D. (2013). Healthcare experiences of autistic adults. *Journal of General Internal Medicine 28*(7), 871. doi:10.1007/s11606-013-2427-z.

Nicolaidis, C., Raymaker, D., Ashkenazy, E., McDonald, K.E. et al. (2015). 'Respect the way I need to communicate with you': Healthcare experiences of adults on the autism spectrum. Autism 19(7), 824–831. doi:10.1177/1362361315576221.

Nicolaidis, C., Raymaker, D., McDonald, K., Dern, S. *et al.* (2012). Comparison of healthcare experiences in autistic and non-autistic adults: A cross-sectional online survey facilitated by an academic-community partnership. *Journal of General Internal Medicine 28*(6), 761–769. doi:10.1007/s11606-012-2262-7.

Nicolaidis, C., Raymaker, D., McDonald, K., Kapp, S. *et al.* (2016). The development and evaluation of an online healthcare toolkit for autistic adults and their primary care providers. *Journal of General Internal Medicine 31*(10), 1180–1189. doi:10.1007/s11606-016-3763-6.

Nicholas, D.B., Zwaigenbaum, L., Muskat, B., Craig, W.R. et al. (2016). Toward practice advancement in emergency care for children with autism spectrum disorder. *Pediatrics 137*(Supplement), S205–S211. doi:10.1542/peds.2015-2851s.

Norton, P.A., Baker, J.E., Sharp, H.C. & Warenski, J.C. (1995). Genitourinary prolapse and joint hypermobility in women. *Obstetrics and Gynecology 85*(2), 225–228.

Nottingham University Hospitals NHS Trust (2023). Services for vulnerable women. www.nuh.nhs.uk/services-for-vulnerable-women.

Nuwer, R. (2015). Body clock genes may set pace for sleep issues in autism. *Spectrum News*, 19 June. www.spectrumnews.org/news/body-clock-genes-may-set-pace-for-sleep-issues-in-autism.

Oakley, A. (1974). *Housewife.* London: Penguin.

Oakley, A. (1979). *From Here to Maternity: Becoming a Mother.* London: Penguin.

Oakley. A. (1984). *The Captured Womb*. Oxford: Basil Blackwell.

O'Connell, M., Martin, C. & Dahlen, H. (2022). Time to rectify past mistakes and take a woman-centred approach to labour progress. *Obstetrics, Gynaecology and Reproductive Medicine 32*(11), 259–261.

O'Driscoll, K., Stronge, J.M. & Minogue, M. (1973). Active management of labour. *British Medical Journal 973*(3), 135–137.

Ogbonnaya, C., Tillman, C.J. & Gonzalez, K. (2018). Perceived organizational support in health care: The importance of teamwork and training for employee well-being and patient satisfaction. *Group & Organization Management 43*(3), 475–503.

Ohlsson Gotby, V., Lichtenstein, P., Långström, N. & Pettersson, E. (2018). Childhood neurodevelopmental disorders and risk of coercive sexual victimization in childhood and adolescence – a population-based prospective twin study. *Journal of Child Psychology and Psychiatry 59*(9), 957–965. doi:10.1111/jcpp.12884.

Øien, R.A., Cicchetti, D.V. & Nordahl-Hansen, A. (2018). Gender dysphoria, sexuality and autism spectrum disorders: A systematic map review. *Journal of Autism and Development Disorders 48*(12), 4028–4037. doi:10.1007/s10803-018-3686-7.

Oliver, D. (2018). David Oliver: NHS workforce policy is not joined-up government. *British Medical Journal 363*, k4417.

Oliver, M. (1997). The social model in context. *Understanding Disability*. doi:10.1007/978-1-349-24269-6_4.

Olthuis, J.V. & Asmundson, G.J. (2019). Optimizing Outcomes for Pain Conditions by Treating Anxiety Sensitivity. In J.A.J. Smits, M.W. Otto, M.B. Powers & S.O. Baird (eds) *The Clinician's Guide to Anxiety Sensitivity Treatment and Assessment* (pp.77–100). Amsterdam: Elsevier Academic Press.

O'Nions, E., Christie, P., Gould, J., Viding, E. & Happé, F. (2013). Development of the 'Extreme Demand Avoidance Questionnaire' (EDA-Q): Preliminary observations on a trait measure for pathological demand avoidance. *Journal of Child Psychology and Psychiatry 55*(7), 758–768. doi:10.1111/jcpp.12149.

Oppenheim, M. (2021). Quarter of parents who suffered domestic abuse say it took place during pregnancy. *The Independent*, 26 February. www.independent.co.uk/news/uk/home-news/domestic-abuse-pregnancy-b1807636.html.

Özçalışkan, Ş., Adamson, L.B. & Dimitrova, N. (2016). Early deictic but not other gestures predict later vocabulary in both typical development and autism. *Autism 20*(6), 754–763.

Parellada, M., Boada, L., Moreno, C., Llorente, C. *et al.* (2013). Specialty care programme for autism spectrum disorders in an urban population: A case-management model for health care delivery in an ASD population. *European Psychiatry 28*(2), 102–109. doi:10.1016/j.eurpsy.2011.06.004.

Parish, S.L., Mitra, M., Son, E., Bonardi, A, Swodoba, P.T. & Igdalsky, L. (2015). Pregnancy outcomes among U.S. women with intellectual and developmental disabilities. *American Journal of Intellectual and Developmental Disabilities 120*(5), 433–443. doi:10.1352/1944-7558-120.5.433.

Patterson, A., Clawson, R., McCarthy, M., Fryson, R. & Kitson, D. (2018). *My Marriage My Choice: Summary of Findings*. University of Nottingham. www.nottingham.ac.uk/research/groups/mymarriagemychoice/documents/summary-full.pdf.

Patterson, J., Hollins Martin, C. & Karatzias, T. (2018). PTSD post-childbirth: A systematic review of women's and midwives' subjective experiences of care provider interaction. *Journal of Reproductive and Infant Psychology 37*(1), 56–83. doi:10.1080/02646838.2018.1504285.

PDA Society (2016). *Diagnosis of PDA: Views of Professionals*. www.pdasociety.org. uk/wp-content/uploads/2019/08/PDA-survey-of-professionals-2016.pdf.

PDA Society (2019). *Being Misunderstood: Experiences of the Pathological Demand Avoidance Profile of ASD*. www.pdasociety.org.uk/wp-content/uploads/2019/08/ BeingMisunderstood.pdf.

PEACE (2020). What is PEACE? https://peacepathway.org.

Pérez D'Gregorio, R. (2010). Special Editorial. Obstetric violence: A new legal term introduced in Venezuela. *International Journal of Gynecology and Obstetrics 111*, 201–202.

Phillips, E. (2019). Autism and pregnancy: A birth experience. The Aspergian. Blog post, 22 April. https://theaspergian.com/2019/04/22/autism-and-birth.

Philpott, R. & Castle, W. (1972). Cervicographs in the management of labour on primigravidae 1. The alert line for detecting abnormal labour. *Journal of Obstetrics and Gynaecology of the British Commonwealth 79*(7), 592–598. doi:10.1111/j.1471-0528.1972.tb14207.x.

Pohl, A.L., Crockford, S.K., Allison, C. & Baron-Cohen, S. (Autism Research Centre, University of Cambridge) (2016). Positive and negative experiences of autistic mothers. Conference presentation at INSAR on 14 May 2016, Baltimore Convention Centre.

Pohl, A.L., Crockford, S.K., Blakemore, M., Allison, C. & Baron-Cohen, S. (2020). A comparative study of autistic and non-autistic women's experience of motherhood. *Molecular Autism 11*, 3. doi:10.1186/s13229-019-0304-2.

Positive Birth Movement & Channel Mum (2016). Birth Survey 2016. www.positivebirthmovement.org/birth-survey-2016.

Potvin, L.A., Brown, H.K. & Cobigo, V. (2016). Social support received by women with intellectual and developmental disabilities during pregnancy and childbirth: An exploratory qualitative study. *Midwifery 37*, 57–64. doi:10.1016/j. midw.2016.04.005.

Preißmann, C. (2017). Autism and healthcare. *Advances in Autism 3*(3), 115–124. doi:10.1108/aia-02-2017-0004.

Price, C., Kantrowitz-Gordon, I. & Calhoun, R. (2019). A pilot feasibility study of mindfulness childbirth education for women with a history of sexual trauma. *Complementary Therapies in Clinical Practice 37*, 102–108. doi:10.1016/j. ctcp.2019.09.005.

Raising Children (2022). Co-occurring conditions and autism. https://raisingchildren.net.au/autism/learning-about-autism/about-autism/conditions-that-occur-with-asd#:~:text=These%20are%20called%20co%2Doccurring,later%20 in%20adolescence%20or%20adulthood.

Rattaz, C., Dubois, A., Michelon, C., Viellard, M., Poinso, F. & Baghdadli, A. (2013). How do children with autism spectrum disorders express pain? A comparison with developmentally delayed and typically developing children. *Pain 154*(10), 2007–2013. doi:10.1016/j.pain.2013.06.011.

Ratto, A.B., Kenworthy, L., Yerys, B.E., Bascom, J. *et al.* (2018). What about girls? Sex-based differences in autistic traits and adaptive skills. *Journal of Autism and Developmental Disorders 48*(5), 1698–1711. doi:10.1007%2Fs10803-017-3413-9.

Redshaw, M., Malouf, R., Gao, H. & Gray, R. (2013). Women with disability: The experience of maternity care during pregnancy, labour and birth and the postnatal period. *BMC Pregnancy and Childbirth 13*, 174. doi:10.1186%2F1471-2393-13-174.

Richards, G., Baron-Cohen, S., Warrier, V., Mellor, B. *et al.* (2022). Evidence of partner similarity for autistic traits, systemizing, and theory of mind via facial expressions. *Scientific Reports 12*(8451).

Rimmer, A. (2016). Why can't the NHS value junior staff the way top companies do? *British Medical Journal 355*(i5740).

Rimmer, A. (2018). Junior doctors' contract: the sticking points in negotiations. *British Medical Journal 352*(i98).

Riquelme, I., Hatem, S.M. & Montoya, P. (2016). Abnormal pressure pain, touch sensitivity, proprioception, and manual dexterity in children with autism spectrum disorders. *Neural Plasticity 2016*, 1–9. doi:10.1155/2016/1723401.

Robbins, L. & Phenicie, B. (2011). Attention deficit hyperactivity disorder and patients with pain. *Practical Pain Management 11*(9).

Roberts, A.L., Koenen, K.C., Lyall, K., Robinson, E. & Weisskopt, M.G. (2015). Association of autistic traits in adulthood with childhood abuse, interpersonal victimization, and posttraumatic stress. *Child Abuse and Neglect 45*, 135–142. doi:10.1016/j.chiabu.2015.04.010.

Roberts, C., Montgomery, E., Richens, Y. & Silverio, S.A. (2023). (Re)activation of survival strategies during pregnancy and childbirth following experiences of childhood sexual abuse. *Journal of Reproductive and Infant Psychology 41*(2), 152–164. doi:10.1080/02646838.2021.1976401.

Roberts, N. (2016). Junior doctor strikes to go ahead after talks collapse. *GP Online*, 4 January. https://www.gponline.com/junior-doctor-strikes-go-ahead-talks-collapse/article/1378089.

Robertson, A.E. & Simmons, D.R. (2015). The sensory experiences of adults with autism spectrum disorder: A qualitative analysis. *Perception 44*(5), 569–586. doi:10.1068/p7833.

Robertson, C.E. & Baron-Cohen, S. (2017). Sensory perception in autism. *Nature Reviews Neuroscience 18*(11), 671–684. doi:10.1038/nrn.2017.112.

Robertson, R., Wenzel, L., Thompson, J. & Charles, A. (2017). *Understanding NHS Financial Pressures: How Are They Affecting Patient Care?* London: The King's Fund.

Robinson, S. & Thompson, A. (1995). *Midwives, Research and Childbirth* (Vol. 4). London: Chapman & Hall.

Rogers, C. (2010). But it's not all about the sex: Mothering, normalisation and young learning disabled people. *Disability & Society 25*(1), 63–74. doi:10.1080/09687590903363365.

Rogers, C., Lepherd, L., Ganguly, R. & Jacob-Rogers, S. (2017). Perinatal issues for women with high functioning autism spectrum disorder. *Women and Birth 30*(2), e89–e95. doi:10.1016/j.wombi.2016.09.009.

Rönnerhag, M., Severinsson, E., Haruna, M. & Berggren, I. (2018). A qualitative evaluation of healthcare professionals' perceptions of adverse events focusing on communication and teamwork in maternity care. *Journal of Advanced Nursing 75*(3), 585–93. doi:10.1111/jan.13864.

Rosen, T.E., Mazefsky, C.A., Vasa, R.A. & Lerner, M.D. (2018). Co-occurring psychiatric conditions in autism spectrum disorder. *International Review of Psychiatry 30*(1), 40–61. doi:10.1080/09540261.2018.1450229.

Ross, L.J. (2018). Reproductive justice as intersectional feminist activism. *Souls: A Critical Journal of Black Politics, Culture, and Society 19*(3), 286–314. doi:10.1080/10999949.2017.1389634.

Roux, A. & Kerns, C. (2016). Awareness, education, and counseling: Supporting mental health for adults with autism. Drexel University, 30 March. https://drexel.edu/autismoutcomes/blog/overview/2016/March/Awareness-Education-and-Counseling-Supporting-mental-health-for-adults-with-autism.

Royal College of Midwives (2016). *State of Maternity Services Report 2016*. London: Royal College of Midwives. www.rcm.org.uk/media/2372/state-of-maternity-services-report-2016.pdf.

Royal College of Midwives (2023). Specialist Mental Health Midwives: What they do and why they matter. www.rcm.org.uk/media/2370/specialist-mental-health-midwives-what-they-do-and-why-they-matter.pdf.

Royal College of Obstetricians and Gynaecologists (2015). Pelvic girdle pain and pregnancy. www.rcog.org.uk/media/e2wouadz/pi-pelvic-girdle-pain-and-pregnancy.pdf.

Ryan, F. (2017). Couples with learning disabilities face unfair wedding bar. *The Guardian*, 30 November. www.theguardian.com/society/2014/jun/17/couples-learning-disabilities-denied-marriage-sexual-relations.

Ryan, F. (2019). Casting a puppet as an autistic child is a grotesque step backwards. *The Guardian*, 12 February. www.theguardian.com/commentisfree/2019/feb/12/casting-puppet-as-autistic-child-step-backwards-new-play-row-other-actors-played-by-humans.

Ryder, L.W. (2017). *Social-Pragmatic Communication in Women with Autism Spectrum Disorder: A Multiple Case Study*. Doctoral dissertation, University of New Hampshire. https://scholars.unh.edu/cgi/viewcontent.cgi?article=1336&context=honors.

Sainsbury, C. (2000). *Martian in the Playground: Understanding the Child with Asperger's Syndrome*. London: SAGE.

Salà, G., Hooley, M., Attwood, T., Mesibov, G. & Stokes, M. (2019). Autism and intellectual disability: A systematic review of sexuality and relationship education. *Sexuality and Disability 37*, 353–382. doi:10.1007/s11195-019-09577-4.

Samadi, S.A. & McConkey, R. (2015). Screening for autism in Iranian preschoolers: Contrasting M-CHAT and a scale developed in Iran. *Journal of Autism and Developmental Disorders 45*(9), 2908–2916.

Samulowitz, A., Gremyr, I., Eriksson, E. & Hensing, G. (2018). 'Brave men' and 'emotional women': A theory-guided literature review on gender bias in health care and gendered norms towards patients with chronic pain. *Pain Research and Management 2018*(3), 1–14. doi:10.1155/2018/6358624.

Sanchez, P. (2018). From 'autism mom' to autistic mother. Autistic Motherland, 21 April. https://americanbadassactivists.wordpress.com/2018/04/21/from-autism-mom-to-autistic-mother-paula-sanchez.

Sarrett, J.C. (2017). Autism and accommodations in higher education: Insights from the autism community. *Journal of Autism and Developmental Disorders 48*, 679–693. doi:10.1007/s10803-017-3353-4.

Sasson, N.J. & Morrison, K.E. (2019). First impressions of adults with autism improve with diagnostic disclosure and increased autism knowledge of peers. *Autism 23*(1), 50–59. doi:10.1177/1362361317729526.

Saunders, N. & Paterson, C. (1991). Can we abandon Naegele's rule? *Lancet 337*(8741), 600–601. 10.1016/0140-6736(91)91653-c.

Sawer, P. (2018a). Autistic woman allowed to have sex with numerous men 'despite not being aware of dangers'. *Daily Telegraph*, 18 October. www.telegraph.co.uk/

news/2018/10/18/autistic-woman-allowed-have-sex-numerous-men-despite-not-aware.

Sawer, P. (2018b). Woman with learning difficulties not told she had contraceptive device covertly fitted. *Daily Telegraph*, 18 October. www.telegraph.co.uk/news/2018/10/18/woman-learning-difficulties-not-told-had-contraceptive-device.

Saxe, A. (2017). The theory of intersectionality: A new lens for understanding the barriers faced by autistic women. *Canadian Journal of Disability Studies 6*(4), 153. doi:10.15353/cjds.v6i4.386.

Schendel, D.D., Overgaard, M., Christensen, J., Hjort, L. et al. (2016). Association of psychiatric and neurologic comorbidity with mortality among persons with autism spectrum disorder in a Danish population. *JAMA Pediatrics 170*(3), 243–250.

Schiller, R. (2019). Was the royal baby really born at home? Here's why I hope you never find out. *The Independent*, 8 May. www.independent.co.uk/news/uk/home-news/royal-baby-meghan-markle-son-home-birth-privacy-rebecca-schiller-a8904341.html.

Schmit, J., Alper, S., Raschke, D. & Ryndak, D. (2000). Effects of using a photographic cueing package during routine school transitions with a child who has autism. *Mental Retardation 38*(2), 131–137. doi:10.1352/0047-6765(2000)038<0131:EOUAPC>2.0.

Schnabel, A. & Bastow, C. (2023). Nothing for us, without us: A review of the clinical literature and discursive evidence of interpersonal trauma in autistic women. *Advances in Autism*. doi:10.1108/AIA-11-2021-0046.

Sedgewick, F., Hull, L. & Ellis, H. (2022). *Autism and Masking: How and Why People Do It, and the Impact It Can Have*. London: Jessica Kingsley Publishers.

Sener, E., Sahin, M., Taheri, S., Bayramov, K. *et al.* (2017). A preliminary study of the genes related with aggression and insensitivity to pain in the autism spectrum disorders. *Bulletin of Clinical Psychopharmacology 1*. doi:10.5455/bcp.20161016114319.

Serafini, G., Gonda, X., Canepa, G., Pompili, M. *et al.* (2017). Extreme sensory processing patterns show a complex association with depression, and impulsivity, alexithymia, and hopelessness. *Journal of Affective Disorders 210*, 249–257. doi:10.1016/j.jad.2016.12.019.

Shakespere, J. (2015). *Practical Implications for Primary Health of the NICE Guideline CG192: Antenatal and Postnatal Mental Health*. London: Royal College of General Practitioners.

Shepherd, J. & Parry, J. (2018). Understanding oral health challenges for children and young people with autistic spectrum conditions: Views of families and the dental team. *Journal of Disability and Oral Health 19*(4), 170–174.

Shield, A. (2014). Preliminary Findings of Similarities and Differences in the Signed and Spoken Language of Children with Autism. *Seminars in Speech and Language 35*(4).

Shkedy, G., Shkedy, D. & Sandoval-Norton, A.H. (2021). Long-term ABA therapy is abusive: A response to Gorycki, Ruppel, and Zane. *Advances in Neurodevelopmental Disorders 5*, 126–134. doi:10.1007/s41252-021-00201-1

Showalter, E. (1987). *The Female Malady: Women, Madness and English Culture 1830–1980*. London: Virgo.

Silberman, S. (2015). *Neurotribes: The Legacy of Autism and How to Think Smarter About People Who Think Differently*. London: Allen & Unwin.

Silberman, S. (2016). Was Dr. Asperger a Nazi? The question still haunts autism. NPR: Health Shots, 20 January. www.npr.org/sections/health-shots/2016/01/20/463603652/was-dr-asperger-a-nazi-the-question-still-haunts-autism.

Singer, J. (1999). 'Why can't you be normal for once in your life?' From a 'problem with no name' to the emergence of a new category of difference. In M. Corker & S. French (eds) *Disability Discourse* (pp.59–67). Buckingham: Open University Press.

Singer, J. (2017). *Neurodiversity: The Birth of an Idea*. Self-published.

Smith, C. (2017). *Understanding Hypermobile Ehlers-Danlos Syndrome and Hypermobility Spectrum Disorder*. Weston-super-Mare: Redcliff-House Publications.

Söderquist, J., Wijma, B. & Wijma, K. (2006). The longitudinal course of post-traumatic stress after childbirth. *Journal of Psychosomatic Obstetrics & Gynecology 27*(2), 113–119. doi:10.1080/01674820600712172.

Somerville, C. (2015). *Unhealthy Attitudes: The Treatment of LGBT People within Health and Social Care Services*. London: Stonewall.

Spain, H. (2022). Mother-led: Reclaiming the childbirth journey. *Midwifery Matters*, September. Association of Radical Midwives.

Sparrow, A. (2015). Why are IFS and Treasury split on who shoulders most of austerity? *The Guardian*, 23 January. www.theguardian.com/business/2015/jan/23/why-ifs-treasury-split-austerity-burden-analysis.

Sperber, D. & Wilson, D. (1986). *Relevance: Communication and Cognition*. Oxford: Blackwell.

Stagg, S.D. & Vincent, J. (2019). Autistic traits in individuals self-defining as transgender or nonbinary. *European Psychiatry 61*, 17–22. doi:10.1016/j.eurpsy.2019.06.003.

Stantić, M., Ichijo, E., Catmur, C. & Bird, G. (2021). Face memory and face perception in autism. *Autism 26*(1). doi:10.1177/13623613211027685.

Stark, E., Ali, D., Ayre, A., Schneider, N. et al. (2021). Coproduction with Autistic Adults: Reflections from the Authentistic Research Collective. *Autism in Adulthood 3*(2), 195–203.

Steenfeldt-Kristensen, C., Jones, C.A. & Richards, C. (2020). The Prevalence of Self-injurious Behaviour in Autism: A Meta-analytic Study. *Journal of Autism and Developmental Disorders 50*, 3857–3873.

Stewart, K. & O'Reilly, P. (2017). Exploring the attitudes, knowledge and beliefs of nurses and midwives of the healthcare needs of the LGBTQ population: An integrative review. *Nurse Education Today 53*, 67–77. doi:10.1016/j.nedt.2017.04.008.

Stilman, J. & Beltramo, J.L. (2019). Exploring Freirean culture circles and Boalian theatre as pedagogies for preparing asset-oriented teacher educators. *Teachers College Record 121*(4). https://eric.ed.gov/?id=EJ1204025.

Strang, J.F., Kenworthy, L., Dominska, A., Sokoloff, J. *et al.* (2014). Increased gender variance in autism spectrum disorders and attention deficit hyperactivity disorder. *Archives of Sexual Behavior 43*(8), 1525–1533. doi:10.1007/s10508-014-0285-3.

Striebich, S., Mattern, E. & Ayerle, G.M. (2018). Support for pregnant women identified with fear of childbirth (FOC)/tokophobia – A systematic review of approaches and interventions. *Midwifery 61*, 97–115. doi:10.1016/j.midw.2018.02.013.

Stubbs, T., Kentikelenis, A., Ray, R. & Gallagher, K.P. (2022). Poverty, inequality, and the International Monetary Fund: How austerity hurts the poor and widens inequality. *Journal of Globalization and Development 13*(1), 61–89.

Studd, J. (1973). Partograms and nomograms of cervical dilatation in management of primigravid labour. *British Medical Journal 4*(5890), 451–455.

Summer, J. & Adavadkar, P. (2023). Autism and Sleep. *Sleep Foundation.* www.sleepfoundation.org/physical-health/autism-and-sleep.

Summers, J., Shahrami, A., Cali, S., D'Mello, C. *et al.* (2017). Self-injury in autism spectrum disorder and intellectual disability: Exploring the role of reactivity to pain and sensory input. *Brain Sciences 7*(11), 140. doi:10.3390%2Fbrainsci7110140.

Suplee, P., Gardner, M., Bloch, J. & Lecks, K. (2014). Childbearing experiences of women with Asperger syndrome. *Journal of Obstetric, Gynecologic and Neonatal Nursing 43*(Suppl 1.), S76. doi:10.1111/1552-6909.12455.

Symon, A. (2017). A case of autism, learning disability, and refusal of planned caesarean. *British Journal of Midwifery 25*(3). doi:10.12968/bjom.2017.25.3.198.

Tavistock and Portman NHS Foundation Trust (2019). Gender identity development services referrals in 2019–20 same as 2018–19. www.tavistockandportman.nhs.uk/about-us/news/stories/gender-identity-development-service-referrals-2019-20-same-2018-19.

Taylor, M. (2014). Caring for a woman with autism in early labour. *British Journal of Midwifery 22*(7), 514–518. doi:10.12968/bjom.2014.22.7.514.

Teixeira, S. & Machado, H. (2016). WHO caesarean section rate: Relevance and ubiquity at the present day – a review article. *Journal of Pregnancy and Child Health 3*(2). doi:10.4172/2376-127x.1000233.

Tek, S., Mesite, L., Fein, D. & Naigles, L. (2014). Longitudinal analyses of expressive language development reveal two distinct language profiles among young children with autism spectrum disorders. *Journal of Autism and Developmental Disorders 44*(1), 75–89.

Thaler, H., Skewes, J.C., Gebauer, L., Christensen, P., Prkachin, K.M. & Jegindø Elmholdt, E. (2017). Typical pain experience but underestimation of others' pain: Emotion perception in self and others in autism spectrum disorder. *Autism 22*(6), 751–762. doi:10.1177/1362361317701269.

The Health Foundation (2016). *Fit for Purpose? Workforce Policy in the English NHS.* London: The Health Foundation.

The Health Foundation (2019). Whorlton Hall abuse scandal. 22 May 2019. https://navigator.health.org.uk/theme/whorlton-hall-abuse-scandal.

Thomas, S., Hovinga, M.E., Rai, D. & Lee, B.K. (2017). Brief report: Prevalence of co-occurring epilepsy and autism spectrum disorder: The US National Survey of Children's Health 2011–2012. *Journal of Autism and Development Disorders 47*(1), 224–229. https://doi.org/10.1007/s10803-016-2938-7.

Tick, B., Bolton, P., Happé, F., Rutter, M. & Rijsdijk, F. (2016). Heritability of autism spectrum disorders: A meta-analysis of twin studies. *Journal of Child Psychology and Psychiatry 57*(5), 585–595. doi:10.1111/jcpp.12499.

Tobia, P. (2017). *The Patients of Bristol Lunatic Asylum in the Nineteenth Century.* PhD thesis, University of West England. https://uwe-repository.worktribe.com/output/887017.

Tommy's (2022). Recurrent miscarriage and being autistic. www.tommys.org/baby-loss-support/stories/miscarriage/recurrent-miscarriage-and-being-autistic.

Tordjman, S., Davlantis, K.S., Georgieff, N., Geoffray, M-.M. et al. (2015). Autism as a disorder of biological and behavioral rhythms: Toward new therapeutic perspectives. *Frontiers in Pediatrics 3*(1).

Turner, E. (2019). Empowering local government or just passing the austerity buck? The changing balance of central and local government in welfare provision in England 2008–2015. *Regional & Federal Studies 29*(1), 45–65.

UNICEF (2019). *UK Baby Friendly Initiative – Theory of Change.* www.unicef.org.uk/babyfriendly/wp-content/uploads/sites/2/2019/04/Baby-Friendly-Initiative-Theory-of-Change.pdf.

UNICEF/NHS (2022). Off to the best start. www.unicef.org.uk/babyfriendly/wp-content/uploads/sites/2/2022/10/Breastfeeding-leaflet.pdf.

University Hospitals of Morecambe Bay NHS Foundation Trust (2023). Our Specialist Midwives. www.uhmb.nhs.uk/our-services/services/maternity-services/our-specialist-midwives.

Van der Gucht, N. & Lewis, K. (2015). Women's experiences of coping with pain during childbirth: A critical review of qualitative research. *Midwifery 31*(3), 349–358. doi:10.1016/j.midw.2014.12.005.

Van Wijngaarden-Cremers, P.J., Van Eeten, E., Groen, W.B., Van Deurzen, P.A., Oosterling, I.J. & Van der Gaag, R.J. (2013). Gender and age differences in the core triad of impairments in autism spectrum disorders: A systematic review and meta-analysis. *Journal of Autism and Developmental Disorders 44*(3), 627–635. doi:10.1007/s10803-013-1913-9.

Verrault, N., Da Costa, D., Marchand, A., Ireland, K. *et al.* (2012). PTSD following childbirth: A prospective study of incidence and risk factors in Canadian women. *Journal of Psychosomatic Research 73*(4), 257–263. doi:10.1016/j.jpsychores.2012.07.010.

Villines, Z. (2023). What is a social battery? Medical News Today, 13 February. www.medicalnewstoday.com/articles/social-battery.

Walsh, K. (2016). Costs and assessment in medical education: A strategic view. *Perspectives on Medical Education 5*(5), 265–267. doi:10.1007/s40037-016-0299-8.

Walsh, K., Levin, H., Jaye, P. & Gazzard, J. (2013). Cost analyses approaches in medical education: There are no simple solutions. *Medical Education 47*(10), 962–968. doi:10.1111/medu.12214.

Ward, J. (2019). Individual differences in sensory sensibility: A synthesising framework and evidence from normal variation and developmental conditions. *Cognitive Neuroscience 10*, 3, 139–157. doi:10.1080/17588928.2018.1557131.

Ward, V. (2018). UK's welfare system is cruel and misogynistic, says UN expert after damning report on poverty. *Daily Telegraph*, 16 November. www.telegraph.co.uk/news/2018/11/16/welfare-system-cruel-misogynistic-un-expert-warns-damning-report.

Watkins, J., Wulaningsih, W., Da Zhou, C., Marshall, D.C. *et al.* (2017). Effects of health and social care spending constraints on mortality in England: A time trend analysis. *BMJ Open 7*(11), e017722. doi:10.1136/bmjopen-2017-017722.

Welsh Government (2019). *Review of Maternity Services at the Former Cwm Taf University Health Board.* www.gov.wales/review-maternity-services-former-cwm-taf-university-health-board.

Whitburn, L.Y., Jones, L.E., Davey, M. & McDonald, S. (2019). The nature of labour pain: An updated review of the literature. *Women and Birth 32*(1), 28–38. doi:10.1016/j.wombi.2018.03.004.

White, E.I., Wallace, G.L., Bascom, J., Armour, A.C. *et al.* (2017). Sex differences in parent-reported executive functioning and adaptive behavior in children and young adults with autism spectrum disorder. *Autism Research 10*, 1653–1662.

Wickham, S. (2021). *In Your Own Time: How Western Medicine Controls the Start of Labour and Why This Needs to Stop.* Avebury: Birthmoon Creations.

Williams, G.L., Wharton, T., & Jagoe, C. (2021). Mutual (mis)understanding: Reframing autistic pragmatic 'Impairments' using relevance theory. *Frontiers in Psychology.* doi: 10.3389/fpsyg.2021.616664.

Williams, S.L. & Mann, A.K. (2017). Sexual and gender minority health disparities as a social issue: How stigma and intergroup relations can explain and reduce health disparities. *Journal of Social Issues 73*(3), 450–461. doi:10.1111/josi.12225.

Willner, P., Scheel-Krüger, J. & Belzung, C. (2014). Resistance to antidepressant drugs: The case for a more predisposition-based and less hippocampocentric research paradigm. *Behavioural Pharmacology 25*(5/6), 352–371. doi:10.1097/FBP.0000000000000066.

Wing, L. (1981a). Language, social, and cognitive impairments in autism and severe mental retardation. *Journal of Autism and Developmental Disorders 11*, 31–44. doi:10.1007/BF01531339.

Wing, L. (1981b). Sex ratios in early childhood autism and related conditions. *Psychiatry Research 5*(2), 129–137. doi:10.1016/0165-1781(81)90043-3.

Wing, L., Gould, J. & Gillberg, C. (2011). Autism spectrum disorders in the DSM-V: Better or worse than the DSM-IV? *Research in Developmental Disabilities 32*(2), 768–773. doi:10.1016/j.ridd.2010.11.003.

Wing, L. & Potter, D. (2002). The epidemiology of autism spectrum disorders: Is the prevalence rising? *Mental Retardation and Developmental Disabilities Research 8*(3), 151–161. doi:10.1002/mrdd.10029.

Wisniewski, D. (2000). *Annual Abstract of Statistics. 2000 Edition, No. 135.* London: The Stationery Office.

Woods, R. (2017). Exploring how the social model of disability can be re-invigorated for autism: In response to Jonathan Levitt. *Disability & Society 32*(7), 1090–1095. doi:10.1080/09687599.2017.1328157.

World Health Organization (WHO) (2017). Determinants of health. https://who.int/news-room/questions-and-answers/item/determinants-of-health.

World Health Organization (WHO) (2018). *WHO Recommendations: Intrapartum Care for a Positive Childbirth Experience.* Geneva: WHO. www.who.int/publications/i/item/9789241550215.

World Health Organization (2019). *International Statistical Classification of Diseases and Related Health Problems*, 11th edn. https://icd.who.int.

Xie, E. & Gemmill, M. (2018). Exploring the prenatal experience of women with intellectual and developmental disabilities: In a southeastern Ontario family health team. *Canadian Family Physician 64*(Suppl. 2), S70–S75.

Yingling, M.E., Hock, R.M. & Bell, B.A. (2018). Time-lag between diagnosis of autism spectrum disorder and onset of publicly-funded early intensive behavioral intervention: Do race–ethnicity and neighborhood matter? *Journal of Autism and Developmental Disorders 48*(2), 561–571. doi:10.1007/s10803-017-3354-3.

Youngson, R. (2008). Compassion in healthcare: The missing dimension of healthcare reform? *Journal of Holistic Healthcare 8*(6), 9.

Yuhas, D. (2019). Untangling the ties between autism and obsessive-compulsive disorder. *Spectrum News*, 27 February. www.spectrumnews.org/features/deep-dive-untangling-ties-autism-obsessive-compulsive-disorder.

Zerbo, O., Massolo, M.L., Qian, Y. & Croen, L.A. (2015). A study of physician knowledge and experience with autism in adults in a large integrated healthcare
system. *Journal of Autism and Developmental Disorders 45*(12), 4002–4014.
doi:10.1007/s10803-015-2579-2.
Zerbo, O., Qian, Y., Ray, T., Sidney, S. *et al.* (2019). Health care service utilization
and cost among adults with autism spectrum disorders in a US integrated
health care system. *Autism in Adulthood 1*(1). doi:10.1089/aut.2018.0004.

Subject Index

Author Index